Epilepsy

A DOCTOR RESPONDS
TO HIS PATIENTS' QUESTIONS

199 Answers
SECOND EDITION

ANDREW N. WILNER MD, FACP

Demos Medical Publishing, 386 Park Avenue South, New York, New York 10016

Library of Congress Cataloging-in-Publication Data

Wilner, Andrew N.
   Epilepsy : 199 answers : a doctor responds to his patients /
by Andrew N. Wilner.— 2nd ed.
     p. ; cm.
Includes bibliographical references and index.
   ISBN 1-888799-70-6 (alk. paper)
  1. Epilepsy—Miscellanea.
  [DNLM: 1. Epilepsy—Popular Works. 2. Epilepsy—Resource Guides.
WL 385 W744ea 2003] I. Title.
  RC372 .W55 2003
  616.8'53—dc21

                                       2002013983

Made in the United States of America

To my mother and father,
for a lifetime of encouragement

—

ACKNOWLEDGMENTS

I WOULD LIKE TO EXPRESS GRATITUDE to my teachers at the Montreal Neurological Institute, in particular Drs. Fred Andermann, Peter Gloor, and Felipe Quesney, for introducing me to the wonderful mysteries of epilepsy and clinical neurophysiology.

The lessons I have learned come from my experience in treating over 1,000 patients with epilepsy. I have tried my best over the years to answer their questions as they have struggled with mine. Any value in this book derives from our work together to control their seizures.

Writing this book would not have been possible without the keen academic atmosphere provided by my partners and colleagues at the Carolinas Epilepsy Center and the support of the staff of Carolina Neurological Clinic, P.A.

The American Epilepsy Society, Epilepsy Foundation, and members of the epilepsy community worldwide provided much valuable resource material.

I have endeavored to make the reference section of this book as complete as possible. These have been updated for this new edition.

I also thank my agent and publisher for their assistance in producing this little book.

And last, but not least, I would like to thank the many thousands of readers who warmly received the first edition of *Epilepsy: 199 Answers,* giving impetus to the creation of this second edition.

PREFACE

WHEN YOU READ *Epilepsy: 199 Answers*, you will learn more about the group of diseases known as epilepsy. You will understand your doctor's language and ask better questions. If you fill in the medical history section, keep your calendar, and carry this book when you visit your doctor, it will help you receive optimal care.

I wrote this book on the premise that accurate and comprehensible medical information can empower epilepsy patients to combat their disease.

To complete the first chapter, "What is Epilepsy?", demanded that I harness all my training and experience. Epilepsy is something different for each one of my patients. For some, it is a rare convulsion, imposing the inconvenience of daily medication and a yearly visit to my office. For others, frequent seizures are part of a devastating constellation of brain injury, mental impairment, and social problems. These patients come to my office accompanied by concerned and often exhausted caregivers, desperately searching for a solution to multiple disabilities of which epilepsy is merely one. In writing this book, I have tried to address the needs of all my patients, whether their epilepsy is mild or severe.

The positive feedback from readers of the first edition of *Epilepsy: 199 Answers* encouraged me to write a new, updated, second edition. Although the principles of epilepsy management have not changed, our sophistication regarding neuroimaging, antiepileptic drugs (AEDs), and surgical treatment has dramatically improved since *Epilepsy:199 Answers* was first published in 1996. It is my hope that anyone with epilepsy, a family member, or health care worker who is searching for information and encouragement regarding epilepsy will find their efforts rewarded within the pages of this book. Both the text and resource sections have been rewritten to reflect the state of the art of epilepsy treatment in 2002.

Since the publication of the first edition of *Epilepsy: 199 Answers*, the US Food and Drug Administration (FDA) has approved four new AEDs; levetiracetam (Keppra®), tiagabine (Gabitril®), oxcarbazepine (Trileptal®), and zonisamide (Zonegran®). Although none of these drugs is a miracle cure, many patients have benefited with fewer seizures or decreased side effects. Another new treatment, the vagal nerve stimulator (VNS), received FDA approval in 1997 and has now been implanted in over 15,000 patients worldwide.

Since 1996, the use of magnetic resonance imaging (MRI) has become much more widespread, leading to more precise diagnoses of the cause of epilepsy in many patients. In particular, mesial temporal sclerosis and neuronal migration disorders are recognized far more frequently. This advance in diagnostic precision has important implications for patient care. Epilepsy due to mesial temporal sclerosis can often be cured by epilepsy surgery, and neuronal migration disorders can have important genetic implications.

Our understanding of the genetic basis of epilepsy continues to grow. In 1996, there were four genes identified responsible for epilepsy syndromes; in 2002 that number has more than doubled to nine. A large research effort is directed to identifying abnormal genes responsible for epilepsy and creating new drugs that target the abnormal products of those genes.

The North American Pregnancy Registry, established in 1996, has enrolled over 2,200 women and begun to publish data regarding the risk of birth defects from various AEDs. A European Pregnancy Registry has also commenced work on this problem. In the years to come, the information gathered by these registries will help guide AED selection for women of childbearing age.

In terms of the place of epilepsy in our society, it is my impression that there is a greater understanding among laypeople about the nature of epilepsy. One piece of evidence to support this feeling is that driving rules in 10 states have been amended, in general enhancing the chances that someone with epilepsy will be able to obtain a driver's license.

Epilepsy: 199 Answers is a valuable tool to help you understand and cope with seizures. Use the resource section that lists the many organizations devoted to helping people with epilepsy. The Epilepsy Foundation, American Epilepsy Society, International Bureau for Epilepsy, International League Against Epilepsy, and many other organizations can help. Seek out a Comprehensive Epilepsy Center if you need one. Relevant phone numbers, addresses, and web sites are listed in the back of the book. Do not hesitate to use them!

The clinical scenarios in this book are based on patients in my own practice. In some cases I have camouflaged the patients a bit, or combined the stories of two patients into one. But these case studies are not imagined or hypothetical; they are real.

A glance at the time line in the front of this book reveals that most of the significant advances in understanding epilepsy have occurred in the last hundred years, many in just the last decade. Modern medicine really can help people with epilepsy. In the twenty-first century, there are more proven treatments for epilepsy than ever before. Work with your doctor and reap the benefits of medical progress. Good luck in taking control of your epilepsy!

TIME LINE

Important Events in the History of Epilepsy

400 BC Hippocrates writes first book on epilepsy, *On the Sacred Disease*

1543 Andreas Vesalius, founder of modern anatomy, publishes *De humani coporis fabrica*

1754 Pedro de Horta writes the first epilepsy textbook in the Western Hemisphere

1857 Charles Locock finds bromide effective for seizure control

1873 Hughlings Jackson correctly defines epilepsy as 'the name for occasional, sudden, excessive, rapid, and local discharges of grey matter'

1886 First successful resective surgery for partial seizures by Victor Horsley

1895 Discovery of x-rays by Konrad Roentgen

1912 Phenobarbital introduced

1921 R. M. Wilder introduces the ketogenic diet as treatment for epilepsy

1929 Hans Berger invents the electroencephalogram

1935 Gibbs, Davis, and Lennox publish the first description of spike and wave discharge from patients with petit mal seizures

1937 Merritt and Putnam demonstrate the antiepileptic action of phenytoin (Dilantin®)

1938 Herbert Jasper organizes a laboratory of electroencephalography at the Montreal Neurological Institute and collaborates with Wilder Penfield, the renowned epilepsy neurosurgeon

1954 Establishment of the American Epilepsy Society, a professional group dedicated to supporting individuals affected by epilepsy through research, education, and advocacy

1968 Establishment of the Epilepsy Foundation, a national voluntary health organization devoted to helping people with epilepsy

1972   Early images of first CAT scanner

1973   Passage of antidiscriminatory Rehabilitation Act

1974   Carbamazepine (Tegretol®) introduced in United States

1975   First comprehensive epilepsy centers established in United States

1978   Valproate (Depakene®) introduced in United States

1980   PET scan identifies epileptic patterns of local cerebral metabolism

1981   MRI introduced into clinical medicine

1988   First vagal nerve stimulator implanted in human being

1990   Passage of the Americans with Disabilities Act

1993   Felbamate (Felbatol®) approved for add-on and monotherapy

1994   Gabapentin (Neurontin®) and lamotrigine (Lamictal®) introduced in United States

1996   Fosphenytoin (Cerebyx®) and topiramate (Topamax®) receive FDA approval

1997   Tiagabine (Gabitril®) and vagal nerve stimulator receive FDA approval

1999   Levetiracetam (Keppra®) receives FDA approval

2000   Oxcarbazepine (Trileptal®) and zonisamide (Zonegran®) receive FDA approval

Contents

ANSWERED QUESTIONS

Chapter 3

AT THE DOCTOR'S OFFICE

Chapter 8

CAN I DRIVE?

Chapter 9

SEIZURES AND WORK

Chapter 10

WOMEN AND EPILEPSY

Chapter 11

My Child with Epilepsy

Chapter 12

Epilepsy and the Elderly

Chapter 13

FIRST AID AND SAFETY TIPS

Chapter 14

CLINICAL RESEARCH: SHOULD I PARTICIPATE IN A DRUG TRIAL?

1. What Is Epilepsy?

Brian handed me his seizure calendar and piled medication bottles on my desk. I picked up his thick chart and asked him how things were going. As I recorded his seizure frequency and drug dosages, a loud wailing sound startled me. I looked up and saw Brian's right arm and leg slowly extend and his whole body stiffen. Then the frightening sound stopped. His eyes closed and he smacked his lips for fifteen seconds. His body relaxed.

After the seizure, Brian was sleepy and confused. I made sure he didn't fall off the chair or wander out of the room. He couldn't answer any questions for about ten minutes. When he became more alert, I told Brian he'd had a seizure.

1. What is epilepsy?

Epilepsy is a brain disorder characterized by recurrent seizures. Some cases of epilepsy are inherited. Scientists have identified nine genes responsible for causing epilepsy.

A variety of insults to the brain can also result in epilepsy, such as a birth defect, a birth injury, a head injury, an infection in the brain, or a brain tumor. In approximately half the cases, a cause cannot be found.

When patients come to me with epilepsy, my job is to try to determine its cause, then to prescribe treatment to control the seizures.

2. What is a seizure?

A seizure is an abnormal electrical discharge of a group of neurons in the brain. Seizures can produce a variety of symptoms, depending on the location of the seizure focus and the spread of the electrical activity through the brain. Here are some examples from patients in my practice:

After a small stroke, my partner's elderly mother experienced minor seizures, which consisted only of a tingling in her right forefinger. Karen has a "funny feeling in my stomach" then becomes confused. Jim has a "vague feeling that I'm losing touch with reality." On one occasion he saw the refrigerator "singing a melody." Alan typically has a feeling that "whatever I am thinking about has happened before" then blacks out. Mary has a feeling that "something isn't right" and her head becomes "numb." She stares, wraps her arms around herself, and rolls up in a ball. Ron has a warning of a "tingling feeling in my mind" followed by loss of consciousness and a fall.

Many of my patients have grand mal convulsions, hard seizures during which they lose consciousness, become stiff, and jerk. Richard only has convulsions twice a year, but when he does they can last for hours. He comes by ambulance to the hospital for an admission to the intensive care unit until we stop the seizures with medications.

Experiencing or watching a seizure can be unsettling. It takes some getting used to.

3. What do I do about a first seizure?

Everyone with a first seizure requires a thorough neurologic evaluation in an attempt to determine the cause of the seizure. All treatment decisions stem from this first evaluation.

Brian's magnetic resonance imaging (MRI) scan revealed that part of his left frontal lobe had not developed properly. This was the cause of his seizures. Another of my patients had a seizure while walking outside to pick up a newspaper. It began with an unpleasant odor. His computed axial tomography (CAT) scan was normal, but the more sensitive MRI revealed a small tumor in his temporal lobe, which we treated with radiation and surgery. A young woman had a seizure while working as a receptionist in a local hotel. Her MRI demonstrated evidence of multiple sclerosis, a relatively uncommon cause of seizures.

4. I've only had one seizure. Do I have epilepsy?

Epilepsy is a clinical condition characterized by recurrent seizures. Technically, you do not have epilepsy if you have only had one seizure. From a practical standpoint, often the results of testing, such as electroencephalography (EEG) and brain imaging, can predict the likelihood of a second seizure and greatly influence whether you need treatment.

Withdrawal from alcohol or addicting drugs can stress the body and cause seizures. If this circumstance is not repeated, the seizure will not recur. This type of provoked seizure is not classified as epilepsy.

5. At what age does epilepsy occur?

Epilepsy can begin immediately after birth or can occur for the first time in old age.

6. Is it contagious?

No.

7. Why me? Why do I have epilepsy?

In order to answer this question, you will probably need to see a neurologist who will ask you many questions and perform a detailed examination of your nervous system. You will have a brain scan (either a computed axial tomography [CAT] or magnetic resonance imaging [MRI] scan) and a brain wave test (electroencephalograph).

In some cases, a treatable cause will be found, such as a brain tumor that can be removed. In others, the cause will be attributed to a past head injury or brain infection. In many patients, no cause will be found. (See Chapters 2 and 3 for more details.)

8. How do I know if it is an epileptic seizure?

Not every spell is an epileptic seizure. Some people faint after donating blood, followed by jerking movements. Others collapse because of an abnormal heart rhythm. People with diabetes can become confused or unresponsive as a result of low blood sugar. Sometimes people pass out under severe emotional stress.

Much of my time at the office and the emergency room is spent determining whether a particular spell was an epileptic seizure, another neurologic or medical disorder, or a psychological problem. Short of recording the event on video and examining the brain waves, the best tool to solve this puzzle is an accurate and detailed account of what actually happened. Take notes if you can and bring a witness with you to the doctor's office.

9. My doctor said I have a seizure disorder. Is that the same thing as epilepsy?

Most likely, yes. In the past, some physicians avoided using the word *epilepsy* in order not to upset patients who mistakenly believed epilepsy to be a mental illness. These misunderstandings are much less common now.

10. My father had complications from cardiac bypass surgery and had his first seizure in the hospital. Does he have epilepsy?

Sometimes people have seizures due to a severe illness, such as pneumonia with kidney and liver problems, or following a difficult operation. In such circumstances, brain dysfunction caused by the illness results in seizures. The seizures disappear when the illness improves. These seizures are not epilepsy.

11. What is the best diagnostic test for epilepsy?

There is no blood test for epilepsy. The most useful test for the neurologist is the electroencephalograph (EEG), which amplifies a patient's brain waves and records them on paper or displays them on a video screen. A typical pattern of spikes occurs during an epileptic seizure. In between seizures, spikes may not be present and the diagnosis can be more difficult. For this reason, multiple EEGs may be needed before a definite diagnosis is made.

Other tests, such as computed axial tomography (CAT scan) and magnetic resonance imaging (MRI), provide a detailed picture of the brain. They can reveal birth defects, tumors, and scars, all of which can cause epilepsy.

Your doctor will diagnose epilepsy based on the findings of the history, physical examination, EEG, and brain scans.

12. How will epilepsy affect my life?

As you can imagine from the previous case histories, epilepsy affects each person differently. For some patients, epilepsy is a childhood condition they outgrow. For others, daily falls and frequent trips to the emergency room for cuts and bruises painfully remind them of the defect in their brain. Seizures restrict driving, work, and social opportunities, and hurt their self-esteem.

Most patients' seizures can be controlled. About half see their seizures disappear with the first medication they try. Others require multiple doctor visits to find the dosage and combination of medications that controls their seizures without intolerable side effects.

A new research drug may be the answer for some patients. Others will stop having seizures only when their seizure focus is surgically removed.

13. What can I do to control my seizures?

Become part of the health care team! The knowledge you gain from reading this book will give you the background to better understand your medical problem and therapeutic options. Filling in the medical history section and seizure calendar in the back of this book will enable you to actively participate in your doctor's decisions about medications and other treatment.

Learn to effectively communicate with your doctor and his staff. They are there to help you. Bring your medications to each doctor visit.

There are three simple things you can do to decrease the severity and frequency of your seizures.

✦ Take your medication regularly. Linking the medication to another routine can help you to remember it. Many of my patients take their medications three times a day, once with each meal. If you take medication twice a day, the first dose can be when you brush your teeth in the morning, the second when you prepare for bed. There are gadgets that can assist you. One of my patients has a watch that beeps when another dose is due. Another has a watch with a voice synthesizer to remind him. Use a pillbox if you need one. You can buy an inexpensive one at a pharmacy.

✦ Get enough sleep! Rob only has seizures when he is sleep-deprived. His seizures are severe and he ends up in the hospital. Once he was almost arrested because his behavior was so bizarre after a seizure.

✦ Follow up regularly with your doctor so that you can work together. If you are having seizures, you need to adjust your dosage or switch to another medication. Make a new appointment each time you leave the office so that the doctor can evaluate your progress.

14. What is intractable epilepsy?

Patients whose seizures recur despite intensive and regular treatment with medications have intractable epilepsy. These patients often resort to new research drugs or seizure surgery because their epilepsy is so difficult to control.

15. Can I die during a seizure?

Death from a seizure is extremely rare, but it can occur. Seizures can cause accidents as well as irregular heart rhythms. In my practice of hundreds of patients with thousands of seizures, two people have died as a direct result of epilepsy. One drowned in a whirlpool at the YMCA (where he should not have gone alone). The other was found in bed, the cause of death probably a heart attack. (See Chapter 13 for epilepsy first aid and tips on accident prevention.) Death can also occur from status epilepticus.

16. What is status epilepticus?

Status epilepticus is a life-threatening condition in which seizures do not stop after 30 minutes or occur one after the other without the patient recovering in between. Prolonged seizures can injure the brain as well as cause heart, lung, and kidney problems. Patients must go to the hospital when they have status epilepticus for treatment with intravenous medication such as diazepam (Valium®), lorazepam (Ativan®), phenytoin (Dilantin®), or phenobarbital. Many cases of status epilepticus can be prevented by making sure antiepileptic medications are taken regularly and in the proper dosage.

2. WHY SO MANY TESTS?

The morning after her senior prom, Pamela fell in the bathroom with her first grand mal convulsion. Her mother called 911 and the ambulance took her to the nearest emergency room. By the time the doctor examined her she was awake, but very tired and complaining of a pounding headache. Her muscles were sore and she had bitten her tongue. Embarrassed to find herself in public dressed only in her nightgown, she wanted to go home. The doctor said she would have to stay in the hospital to have an electroencephalogram (EEG) and a magnetic resonance imaging (MRI) scan.

17. What is an EEG?

An EEG machine, or electroencephalograph, records electrical activity from your brain. Electrodes are glued or pasted to the scalp and the machine is turned on. Amplifiers magnify the brain's tiny electrical signals. These are usually written on large pieces of paper by sensitive pens. The brain waves can also be digitized and viewed on a computer monitor. A distinctive electrical pattern called "spike and wave" often occurs in patients with epilepsy. Other abnormalities, such as "slow waves," may indicate areas of the brain that fail to function optimally.

18. What is the purpose of an EEG?

Pamela needs an EEG because this is her first seizure. If her EEG is normal, her doctor may choose not to give her any medication, hoping that the seizure was caused by a late night out (sleep deprivation) and possibly some alcohol. On the other hand, if there is a lot of epileptic activity, her risk of a second seizure is high.

Additionally, the pattern of spike and wave will define the seizure type. (Is the epileptic activity limited to one region of the brain, or is it widespread? Is there more than one focus?) Determining the exact type of epilepsy will help her doctor prescribe the medication most likely to control her seizures.

19. Why do I have to stay up all night before my EEG?

Sometimes your doctor will order a "sleep-deprived EEG." Fatigue tends to bring out the worst in brain waves. Most patients with epilepsy learn that sleep deprivation increases their chances of having a seizure. That is why under normal circumstances adequate rest is so important. By having you stay up all night, your doctor is maximizing the chance that epileptic activity will appear on the tracing. This information will guide his choice of medication or help predict the likelihood of a seizure recurrence.

20. Why do they flash a bright light in your eyes during an EEG?

About 5 percent of people with seizures have "photosensitive epilepsy." In these patients, flashing lights can trigger a seizure. Seizures can occur from strobes, television screens, or computer games. Sometimes the flashing light during the EEG, called "photic stimulation," causes spike and wave to appear or even causes a seizure. This clinches the diagnosis. (One of my photosensitive patients had her first convulsion while riding in a car and looking out the window at a forest. The sunlight flashing between the trees provoked a grand mal convulsion. Luckily, she was in the back seat!)

21. Why do I have to hyperventilate during the EEG?

During an EEG, you may be asked to deep breathe for three to five minutes. For reasons that are not completely understood, hyperventilation lowers the seizure threshold and can bring out epileptic activity. In some patients, the EEG changes dramatically during hyperventilation, revealing more about the inner workings of the brain.

22. I already had one EEG. Why do I have to get another?

An EEG records twenty minutes of brain activity. A patient always has abnormal brain waves during a seizure, but brain waves may be normal between seizures. Your doctor may order several EEGs in order to get a good look at the brain waves. I had one patient who had five normal EEGs before we finally found the epileptic activity in her right temporal lobe.

23. Is there any danger when I'm hooked up to the EEG machine?

An EEG is completely safe because the EEG records the brain's own electricity.

24. If I've had an EEG, why do I have to have an MRI?

An EEG is the best way to find out about brain waves, but it does not tell much about the structural anatomy of the brain. For example, slow waves in the left temporal lobe on EEG may be the result of an old head injury. On the other hand, a brain tumor could cause the same type of slowing. Clearly, the treatment for these two problems is different. Whereas no treatment might be needed for the head injury, a brain tumor might require an operation or radiation therapy.

In order to determine the cause of the abnormal EEG, your doctor needs an accurate picture of your brain. The MRI or CAT (computerized axial tomography) scan are two excellent ways to see inside the brain.

25. What is the difference between an MRI and a CAT scan?

Both are new technologies. The CAT scan was the first x-ray machine to rely heavily on the computer, taking thousands of images and reconstructing them into a picture of the brain. The MRI also uses a computer, but employs a strong magnetic field instead of x-rays. CAT scans are quicker and often better for head injuries. MRI scans show more detail.

Epilepsy specialists use the MRI to look for subtle abnormalities in the brain that can cause seizures. One of my patients with terrible memory problems had a normal CAT scan, but his MRI revealed scarring of his left temporal lobe. This lesion was probably the cause of his seizures and memory difficulty.

26. I've been seizure-free for four years and want to stop my medication. Why does my doctor want to do another EEG?

It is extremely difficult to predict seizure recurrence. The fact that you have done well for four years is encouraging. You are probably driving and working. Your doctor is concerned you may have a seizure when you go off medications. Your medical history, seizure type, findings on neurologic exam, brain imaging, and EEG all go into the equation to estimate the risk of seizure recurrence.

Most neurologists believe that it is wise to continue medication if signs of epilepsy persist on the EEG. This has been my experience as well. By repeating your EEG, your doctor is trying to help you make an informed decision. If your EEG is completely normal, he will probably agree to decrease the dose with the goal of discontinuing the medication. (As a precaution against a possible seizure, for the first few weeks after stopping your medication, you may wish to limit driving and avoid potentially dangerous activities such as riding a bicycle, working at heights, and swimming.)

3. AT THE DOCTOR'S OFFICE

Everything was fine when Sally went to bed Sunday night. The next day at the office, she collapsed. Her coworkers said she let out a strange sound, fell off her chair, and jerked. She woke up in the emergency room (ER) with a throbbing headache and a sore tongue. A nurse drew her blood. Then she had an electrocardiogram (EKG) and a computed axial tomography (CAT) scan. The doctor said all the tests were normal and sent her home.

On Tuesday morning Sally was supposed to represent her department at an important meeting. Instead, she was sitting in my waiting room waiting for her appointment. Sally tried to read her typed notes but couldn't concentrate.

What was the neurologist going to do, she wondered? What was wrong with her? It was a question of epilepsy, that's what the emergency room doctor said. Whatever it was, she didn't want it to happen again. How could she help the neurologist figure it out?

27. What should I expect when I go to the neurologist for the first time?

Before the visit with the doctor, you will be asked to complete a screening questionnaire. You will need to list any operations you may have had, medical problems, medications, allergies, habits (like smoking and alcohol), and any illnesses in your family. Most people need to consult with other family members to get all of this information correct. It is best to review your medical history with your parents or spouse before you go to the doctor. Use the guide in Appendix A to prepare this information.

Here are some examples of important questions you might ask them: Were there any problems when I was born? How old was I when I learned to walk and talk? Was it my aunt or uncle who had seizures? Did I ever have a head injury as a child? Wasn't there some medication they gave me in the hospital when I had a broken leg that made me sick to my stomach? Learning the answers to these questions ahead of time will make the completed questionnaire more valuable to your doctor.

Additionally, there will be administrative paperwork to complete before you see the doctor. You will need to provide the name of your insurance plan if you have one. The easiest way to do this is to bring your insurance card. You will also be asked to write down your name, address, phone number, family doctor's name, and other basic information. Include a phone number of a family member or someone close to you whom you would want called if you become seriously ill.

28. What will the doctor do?

Your neurologist will begin with what doctors call a "history and physical." First, he will ask questions about your medical past to try to determine if there is an underlying cause for your seizures. For example, did you ever have a head injury, a family history of epilepsy, encephalitis, or meningitis? He will ask about your general state of health and medications to see whether these factors may have provoked a seizure. He will ask you to describe what you felt when you had the seizure. Some patients experience a warning, or "aura," which often is quite an unusual feeling.

When your doctor is satisfied that he has learned everything he can from talking with you, he will perform a thorough neurologic examination. He will look into your eyes with a bright light, tap your reflexes, ask you to walk, maybe even hop. He will ask you to touch your finger to your nose and smile. Some of the things he asks you to do may seem odd. The neurologic examination is the most lengthy and complex of all medical examinations. Its purpose is to complete a functional inventory of the entire nervous system. It took me over a year to learn to do it when I was a neurology resident, and I am still finding ways to do it better.

At the end of the visit the doctor will explain to you what he thinks the problem is. He may defer making a diagnosis until he has the results of more tests, such as an electroencephalogram (EEG) or magnetic resonance imaging (MRI). He may write a prescription for antiepileptic medication. The doctor will explain to you the dosage and likely side effects. In most cases, you will need to return within a few weeks for a follow-up visit.

29. How long will the visit take?

For your first meeting with a neurologist, expect to spend approximately one hour with the doctor. Plan to arrive at least thirty minutes ahead of time to complete the paperwork before seeing the doctor.

30. Is there anything I should bring?

All your old records. In Sally's case, one hopes that the emergency room doctor faxed the records to the doctor's office. If she had had a chance, it would have been worthwhile for her to go to the hospital and get her CAT scan and a copy of her ER sheet to bring with her.

If you have had epilepsy for a long time and have been treated by other physicians, try to make sure those records get to your new doctor before you do. That way, your doctor will have an opportunity to review them before your visit. If you have had x-rays or EEGs, he will need these results as well. You can help a great deal in the process. I would suggest the following:

+ Write a letter to your previous doctor requesting that all records, x-rays, and EEG reports be mailed to your new doctor. Provide the address. Your letter will serve as a written release. A phone call is not sufficient. Because your medical records are confidential, they cannot be forwarded without your written consent.

   Do not be embarrassed that you are changing doctors. New patients come to me all the time from other doctors. Sometimes patients switch because they are new in town. In other instances, patients are not satisfied with their current doctor. (If you are not getting along with your doctor, you will probably both benefit from a change.)
+ Stop by the hospital or imaging center where your x-rays were done and get a copy of the films. Mail them to your new doctor or bring them to his office before your first appointment.
+ Call your new doctor's office a week before your appointment and check to see whether the old records arrived. If they have not, call your previous doctor and make sure they have been sent. Pick them up in person if you can.
+ Send a written request to any hospital where you have been admitted for your seizures so that these records are forwarded as well.

All these steps may sound like a lot of work, but they are often necessary to make sure the records get where they need to go. The technology of medical record keeping has lagged behind the dramatic advances in other areas of medicine. With the exception of the fax machine, medical records are still transferred the old-fashioned way, by mail or on foot.

(Don't do what some patients do. They either arrive without records ever being sent or on the day of their appointment they carry in with them piles of x-rays and pounds of photocopied pages from three different doctors, drop them on my desk, and ask, "Well, doctor, what do you think?")

In order to render a useful opinion in a complicated case, I will often spend over an hour reading a patient's chart. Then I take the x-rays to the hospital and review them with the neuroradiologist, which takes another thirty minutes to an hour. If the case is unusual, I may need to look something up in a textbook or medical journal, requiring another hour or so. Although I might like to, my schedule won't permit me to spend three hours reviewing records and reading a textbook during a patient visit.

On the other hand, when I do receive all the old records before a patient comes, that first visit becomes much more exciting. I am looking forward to seeing the patient to fill in the gaps in the story. I know what has been done and how well it has been done. I know what stones still need to be turned. If I need to review the medical literature, I can do it ahead of time and be fully prepared for that new patient. My history and physical examination can be very directed, and a plan of action rapidly constructed. These patients get off to a running start.

31. What if he asks me questions I can't (or don't want to) answer?

It always pays to be completely frank with your doctor. If you do not know whether you had febrile seizures as a child, say so. Few patients know the answers to every question. Just do your best.

On the other hand, do not withhold information. For example, if the doctor asks if you drink alcohol, don't say "no" if the answer is "yes." Alcohol abuse is often associated with seizures, and it may be the cause of your problem. Misleading the doctor will result in unnecessary tests and possibly inappropriate medication, and will not help you get rid of the seizures.

An interesting story: I had two patients in the hospital with positive drug screens for marijuana. They both claimed they do not smoke the drug, but their friends do. They wanted me to believe the marijuana got into their system by passive smoking. Possible? Yes. Likely? No. Bite the bullet and tell the truth. Everything you say is confidential. Remember, your doctor is there to help you.

32. Can I bring anyone with me?

Absolutely! Bring someone with you, not only to the doctor's office, but into the examining room. This can be a family member or close friend. Although you may be embarrassed to have someone else bear witness to your illness, that person can help you a great deal. If you can, bring someone who has seen your seizures.

Research into the doctor–patient relationship confirms that few patients remember everything that their doctor says. Many do not recall even half of what they are told. This difficulty in communication is a problem for doctors and patients in every medical field. Doctors sometimes use language that patients cannot understand, and patients are often so anxious they do not remember what was said.

To further complicate the situation, epilepsy patients often have memory impairment, which makes it even more difficult for them to remember instructions accurately. Your companion is likely to be much calmer and more relaxed than you. You will have two sets of ears instead of one, and another mouth to ask questions.

33. How can I remember all my questions?

It pays to bring a list. Try to prioritize; give your doctor an opportunity to answer the most important questions. If you have a question about an article you read in a newspaper or magazine, bring it with you for your doctor to look at. I remember one patient who told me about a promising new treatment he had read about, but could not remember its name. We wasted a fair amount of time trying to figure out what it was. My patient was quite disappointed in me, certain he was missing out on a medical breakthrough. When he finally brought in the article, it was a medication I was already aware of, and it was not appropriate for him. We could have spent that time much more productively discussing the results of his electroencephalogram (EEG) and exploring the possibility of epilepsy surgery.

34. How can I remember all the answers?

Whenever I make any changes in medication, I give my patients my business card with written instructions on the back. If they have any questions, they can call me. When your doctor writes a new prescription, the dosage will be typed on the bottle. A few of my patients have brought tape recorders to the office to record our conversation. I discourage this practice, as it is rarely necessary.

If you are not sure what your doctor said, ask him to repeat it or write it down. Following instructions is important. In a recent survey of over 800 physicians, 92 percent of them felt that compliance was an issue with their epilepsy patients.

35. Why doesn't my doctor spend more time with me?

Although the time with your doctor may be brief, one of the advantages of an office visit is that the physician's total focus will be on you. An office visit is an intimate experience—just you, a family member or close friend, and your doctor. In my office, there are no telephones in the examining room, and interruptions are limited to emergencies. Although there are many tasks competing for the doctor's time in a busy office, the time you spend in the examining room is completely devoted to your care. A great deal can be accomplished during this "quality time."

Depending on complexity, a follow-up visit takes between five and thirty minutes. This is "face to face" time with the physician. It does not include the hours your doctor may have spent reviewing your records and x-rays, or obtaining history or other information from a referring physician or family members.

If you think you need more time with your doctor, say so. If your case is complex and there are things you do not understand, tell your doctor that you would like a longer visit. I sometimes schedule a family conference when a patient's case is difficult or they are not doing well. This provides adequate time for everyone to ask questions and thoroughly understand the problems and the options for treatment.

36. Why is my doctor always late?

I schedule new patients for an hour and follow-up patients for fifteen minutes. Sometimes I finish a new patient in forty-five minutes; sometimes it takes an hour and a half. A follow-up can be as brief as five minutes or as long as thirty minutes. The plan is for it all to equal out by the end of the day. Sometimes it works, but frequently the plan fails. I run late. I don't like it, but it happens. I don't want to rush through anyone's visit, and if new problems come up, they need to be addressed. I would much prefer to finish on time.

I remember one patient who was angry with me because I was an hour late for his appointment. Unfortunately, he didn't tell me. He was sullen during the visit and didn't tell me much about his problems with his seizures. At the end of the visit, he suddenly began to rant and rave about how inconsiderate I was to waste his valuable time. It was late in the afternoon on a busy day, and I didn't even know I was behind schedule. I wish he had told me sooner so I could have apologized and gotten on with the visit. As it was, we didn't accomplish much and neither one of us was very happy. (Listening to him complain took even more time, and my next patient wasn't happy either.)

The busier your doctor is, the more likely he will be off schedule. It is best to prepare for this. Assume he will be late. Bring a book or office paperwork with you to your appointment. If you can, leave children at home with a babysitter or friend. Trying to control energetic kids in a busy waiting room can be fatiguing.

If your doctor tends to run late, there is something you can do. Explain to the scheduling secretary that this is a problem for you and ask for the earliest appointment in the morning or the first one after lunch. Your doctor is more likely to be prompt for these appointments. If that doesn't help, you might check around for another doctor!

37. What do I need to bring to a follow-up visit?

In order to help you manage your seizures, there is a minimum of information your doctor needs at every visit. He needs to know your history and findings of your physical and neurologic examination, as well as results of any testing you may have had, such as MRI or EEGs. All of this information has already been collected during your initial consultation and will be in your chart.

You need to provide two additional pieces of information at each visit. First is the number of seizures you have had. I recommend a seizure calendar. I give each patient a seizure calendar that is good for six months, but you can use any kind of calendar you want. (There is one in Appendix A). I have very few patients who can recall how many seizures they have had without writing them down. And remember, it doesn't do the doctor any good if you keep a seizure calendar and leave it stuck on the refrigerator! (I heard that one yesterday.) Bring it with you. Second, your doctor needs to know which medication you are taking and the correct dose. The easiest thing to do is to bring the bottles with you.

38. How can I get the most out of an office visit?

First of all, don't be late. The time reserved for you will disappear if you are not there. If your doctor has other appointments following yours, your visit will likely be cut short.

If you have small children, find someone to look after them while you are with the doctor. You won't be able to pay attention to a crying baby and your doctor's technical explanation about your seizures at the same time!

Because time with your doctor is limited, it is critical to know how to use it to your advantage. The worst thing you can do is wait for the visit to be nearly over, then tell the doctor that you have just started getting these terrible headaches, or pull out a list of things that have been bothering you. If you present your doctor with a new complaint, he will likely have to perform a more extensive examination than he was anticipating. A complete neurologic examination can take fifteen minutes or a lot longer, depending on the problem and the patient. He may also have to review your chart, looking for similar symptoms you may have had in the past. Again, this will take time. Most medical records are not computerized and it can take many minutes to locate information in a thick chart.

If you wait until the end of your visit to get to the real reason why you are there, you have placed your doctor in an impossible position. If he is like me, there is a waiting room full of patients and he doesn't want to apologize to them for the rest of the day because he is running late. On the other hand, in order to treat your new problem appropriately, he will need to review your chart and perform a neurologic examination. He wants to take proper care of everyone, and now he's in a bind.

When you see your doctor, say hello, then tell him why you are there. For example, "Doctor, I haven't seen you for six months, and I'm here for a check-up." Or, "Doctor, I saw you three months ago but that medicine doesn't really agree with my stomach, and my seizures are no better." Better yet, "Doctor, that new medication I started yesterday gave me a rash, so I came right in. Take a look at these welts!" If you can help your doctor focus on your problem, you will get the best advantage of his time and skill. He will appreciate your forthrightness and you will get a better result. Teamwork with your doctor is your goal.

39. Why do I have to bring my medication with me if the doctor has all the information in the chart?

I used to wonder this myself. Interestingly, there are many variables that determine which medication and how much a patient actually takes. Although I record this information in each patient's chart at every visit, it never ceases to amaze me how often what I have written down does not agree with what the patient tells me at the next visit. I have learned from experience that there are a number of situations that can cause this problem:

+ The patient does not understand verbal instructions. This happens from time to time. Now, when I make a change in dosage or medication, I write it down and hand it to the patient. This usually works.
+ Second, there was confusion over dosing. Many pills come in different strengths. Divalproex sodium (Depakote®), for example, comes in 250 mg and 500 mg sizes. I have had quite a few patients who did not know which dose they were on. One patient knew she was taking five pills but for months we could never determine whether she was taking 1,250 mg or 2,500 mg. Even though the pills are different colors, we still could not figure it out! (This became a problem when she needed a refill.)
+ Sometimes the dosage is adjusted over the phone between visits.

Although these changes are supposed to be entered into the chart, this does not always happen. One reason is that sometimes the change is made by another physician. This may happen over the phone at night when the chart is not available, or during a visit to the hospital or emergency room.

✦ The patient is not taking the prescribed dosage because the prescription was not filled properly. Mistakes by a pharmacist are rare. More frequently, certain pills are not available, such as the 30 mg size phenytoin (Dilantin®), and the prescription isn't filled.

✦ The patient tried the new dose, but developed symptoms of toxicity and went back to the old dose without telling the doctor. This happens all the time. If you need to make a change, inform your doctor. Don't wait until the next visit to tell him you're not doing what he thinks you're doing. Remember that communication is essential to cooperation.

Bringing your medication with you also allows your doctor to see which drugs have been prescribed by other physicians. Some of these may interact with the ones you are taking or with one he is thinking of prescribing. When you bring your bottles with you, it provides a double check to ensure that both you and your doctor know the type and dose of your medication. Don't leave home without them!

40. I keep running out of medication and have to call the office for a refill. I seem to spend a lot of time "on hold." What can I do?

In order to refill a prescription over the phone, your chart has to be pulled by someone in medical records and reviewed by the doctor, and the pharmacy has to be called. If the doctor is at the hospital or with patients, he will not be able to attend to it right away. If you have recently been seen in the office, your chart is likely being typed and may be difficult to locate.

The best thing to do is to check how much medication you have left before you visit the doctor. It is much easier for him to write a refill prescription while you and your chart are together. At each office visit I try to ask patients if they need a refill, but I don't always remember. If you do need a new prescription, it is preferable to call during business hours. Some patients seem to think they cannot refill their prescription until there are absolutely no pills left in the bottle. (This is not true.) Then they call at midnight, desperate because they have run out. Try to avoid this awkward situation by planning ahead. Your doctor will appreciate it.

41. Is there anyone besides my doctor who can explain things to me?

Your doctor will try to answer questions about your disease, tests, and medications. Some questions, such as how to obtain assistance in purchasing medication or arranging transportation, may be better answered by a social worker or nurse. You and your family may benefit from an instructional videotape or epilepsy support group. In-depth information can be found in several excellent books and educational pamphlets listed in the catalog of the Epilepsy Foundation.

If you think you need more information, ask your doctor to refer you to an epilepsy center where many of these services will be available to you. There are over 50 epilepsy centers in the United States that specialize in the treatment of patients with difficult to control seizures. (See Appendix D.)

42. I have several doctors. How can I make sure they are all working together?

In these days of specialized medical care, many patients have two or more physicians. In fact, all of my patients have a primary care physician. Some patients even have other neurologists in their hometowns. A large number of my patients see psychiatrists, who also prescribe medication, typically for depression or anxiety. (These are common problems in patients with epilepsy.)

When a patient's case is complex, I make sure that a copy of my note is sent to the other doctors involved. This can be facilitated if you bring the business cards of your other doctors with you, so the name and address is clear. (I sometimes have patients who request that their notes be sent to their other neurologist, but they don't know who he is!) Remember, good communication leads to good results.

4. MEDICATIONS

For the last three months, Gloria's seizures had gone out of control. She dutifully recorded each one in her calendar and telephoned me every month. With each call, I increased the dose of her medication by one-half a tablet. A week ago, she ran out of medication and refilled her prescription at a new pharmacy close to home.

Today, she sat in my office as an emergency work-in; she was so dizzy she could barely walk. She couldn't focus her eyes and felt sick to her stomach. I opened her chart to see which medication she was taking and asked her the dose. She couldn't remember, so I asked to see the bottle.

When Gloria pulled the plastic bottle out of her purse, she squirmed in her chair. She knew I had told her to take the brand name medication, not the generic. But the brand name was too expensive, she thought, almost fifty cents a pill, and she had to take six of them a day! She couldn't afford it, but was too embarrassed to say anything.

When I saw that the bottle contained round white pills, not the thin pink ones, I confronted her. Didn't she know her seizure disorder was too severe to expect successful treatment with a generic? Why hadn't she followed instructions?

Despite her blurred vision, Gloria could see I was frustrated and annoyed. She began crying and stumbled out of the room. She told herself she'd have to find a better doctor, one who was more sympathetic and could really help with her seizures. Initially, I was perplexed. Why didn't Gloria follow instructions?

43. Why should I take the brand name medication if the generic contains the same active ingredient and costs less?

Sometimes generic medication is adequate. However, it may not be appropriate for patients with difficult to control seizures. Although the active ingredient in each pill or capsule may be identical to the brand name preparation, the amount of medication absorbed and the rate at which it is taken up by the body may not be the same. (The Food and Drug Administration allows a difference of up to 20 percent in bioequivalence from the brand name preparation.)

Additionally, one generic preparation is not identical to another. This variability between brands may be the reason Gloria became toxic on her medication. The last batch of pills she bought at the new pharmacy happened to be better absorbed and gave her a higher drug level.

Patients whose seizures respond easily to medication do not require frequent dosage adjustments and constant drug levels are less critical. In more difficult to control patients, small differences in bioavailability can be more significant. When patients suffer persistent seizures, I recommend brand name medication so that we have a better chance to obtain consistent, effective blood levels.

Had Gloria brought her husband with her, he could have explained that she was taking the generic medication because of financial constraints. He would have calmed her down, and the office visit could have turned into a productive one.

44. My doctor keeps writing prescriptions for these new epilepsy drugs, but I can't afford them! What can I do?

Based on my experience, your doctor is probably preoccupied with the complex medical decision making required to treat your epilepsy rather than thinking about whether you can actually afford the medication.

Of course, both are important. One of my patients told me he was taking a dose lower than I had prescribed because of "side effects." When I pressed him for details, he eventually admitted the drug was too expensive and he couldn't pay for the full dose.

If you cannot afford the prescribed medication, tell your doctor. There are a number of ways he may be able to help you:

+ He may have free samples that can get you started for several days. If you do not tolerate the medication, at least you will not have invested money for a whole month's supply.
+ He may be able to enroll you in a "patient assistance program." Many patients with epilepsy have difficulty buying medication. Because of this problem, most manufacturers of antiepileptic drugs provide medication at no charge for a limited time. Eligibility is determined by the company. A specific form must be completed by your physician and sent to the pharmaceutical company to enroll you in the program. (I fill out many of these forms every month.)

✦ Your doctor can refer you to a social worker who may find other forms of financial support for you, such as Medicare or Medicaid. Many of my patients receive financial assistance.

✦ He can change the prescription to a low cost drug such as phenobarbital if he thinks it will be sufficiently effective.

✦ Join a local epilepsy support group. Remember, you are not alone. Epilepsy is a common disorder, affecting almost 1 percent of the population. Chances are other members of the support group have already located the pharmacies in town with the best prices.

45. Why does epilepsy medication cost so much?

It is hard to imagine a tiny pill being worth one or two dollars. This adds up to a lot of money if you take many of them each day. In my research in drug development, I have had the opportunity to work closely with pharmaceutical companies that manufacture antiepileptic drugs. Each new drug must be shown to be safe and effective before it can be approved by the Food and Drug Administration (FDA). (See Chapter 14.)

Most experimental drugs never succeed in reaching the marketplace, driving up the cost of the ones that do. It takes ten to fifteen years of work by clinical investigators and between three and four hundred million dollars to bring a new drug to market. The price of the drug reflects these high developmental costs.

46. What is the best drug for seizure control?

When I prescribe a new antiepileptic medication, I have to choose the appropriate drug for the seizure type, decide whether it will be used alone (monotherapy) or in combination with other antiepileptic drugs (polytherapy), consider possible drug interactions, estimate the right dose for the patient's body size and metabolism, and devise an easily tolerated dosing schedule.

There are more than a dozen commonly used antiepileptic drugs. (See Appendix B for generic and brand names.) The best drug for seizure control is the one that stops your seizures with the lowest dose and causes the fewest side effects.

47. What do I do if I forget a dose of medication?

In general, my advice is to make it up. Otherwise it may take several days for your drug level to return to normal. However, if your next dose is due within the next hour or two, you are likely to develop toxic symptoms (nausea, dizziness) if you take the pills so close together. In that case, it's better to resume your schedule and make up the missed dose 3 to 4 hours after your next dose.

If you frequently forget your medication, there are techniques to help you remember. Try taking your medication at specific times of day, or in conjunction with certain activities (i.e., breakfast, brushing your teeth, going to bed). Alarms, pill boxes, and other devices may help. (See Question #13).

48. Why do I have to get antiepileptic drug levels?

Because of difference in body size and metabolism, it is difficult to know which dose to prescribe for each patient. Drug levels allow the doctor to monitor how much drug is in your system at a given time.

When one of my patients has a seizure, I often order a drug level. I increase the dose if the level is low. If, on the other hand, the level is high, I am more inclined to switch to a different medication.

When patients complain of symptoms such as dizziness or clumsiness, I order a drug level to see whether the medication is responsible. If the level is high, I lower the dose and wait for the patient to improve. If the level is low, the patient's symptoms are likely due to another neurologic problem that requires further investigation.

Drug levels are also a useful way to monitor compliance. Jan complained of daily seizures despite a combination of phenytoin (Dilantin®) and divalproex sodium (Depakote®). When I checked the levels of these drugs in her blood, both were zero! It didn't take a medical degree to figure out why the medications were not working.

49. Why do I have to take medication three times a day?

The purpose of spreading doses throughout the day is to maintain a constant blood level. After you swallow a pill, your body absorbs it and proceeds to break it down and excrete it. The speed of this process varies in different people.

Additionally, some medications last longer in the body than others. Phenobarbital, for example, is metabolized slowly; it can be taken in one daily dose. Carbamazepine (Tegretol®) is metabolized more rapidly, and ideally should be taken three times a day.

The more difficult the seizures are to control, the more important it is to maintain a steady blood level throughout the day. Frequent doses of medication can improve seizure control.

50. My medication dose keeps increasing. Am I becoming immune to my medication?

A phenomenon called "autoinduction" can occur with some antiepileptic drugs, particularly carbamazepine (Tegretol®). In essence, the body learns to metabolize the drug more effectively. Consequently, a higher dose may be required to maintain the same drug level after several months of use.

51. Will I have to take this medication forever?

Many children outgrow their epilepsy and will no longer require medication. Some adults become seizure-free after their first or second seizure and their medication can often be successfully discontinued. On the other hand, if you are an adult and have had seizures for many years, you will probably do worse without medication.

With continued medical progress, more effective treatments with fewer side effects will likely become available in the future.

5. MEDICATION SIDE EFFECTS

A week after I prescribed a new medication for Janet, she called the office. I had warned her that a rash was one of the potential side effects of this new antiepileptic medication, and now she had one. Her husband had noticed large, red blotches on her back. I asked her to come to the office so that I could see it.

Upon examination that afternoon, I found three saucer-shaped areas on her back about five inches in diameter. There were none on her face, chest, or arms. This was not a typical drug reaction. I sent her to the dermatologist to be sure.

Janet was happy with the cream the dermatologist gave her. After a week of applying the medicine four times a day, the rash went away. It seems she had a fungal infection on her back, something like athlete's foot. I didn't have to change her antiepileptic medication and her seizures have been controlled.

52. What else can cause a rash besides a new drug?

In Janet's case, it was a fungal infection. I remember one patient who complained of a rash on his legs after he began a new medication; he turned out to have flea bites. Another patient complained of a rash on her face, which was adolescent acne. I used to assume that all rashes were related to medications, but now I insist on seeing the patient before I make changes in therapy.

53. What should I do if I break out in a rash?

Call your doctor immediately. In many cases, your doctor will ask you to stop the medication as the rash may represent an allergic reaction. In certain circumstances, your doctor may wish to continue the medication. I usually ask my patients to come to the office so that I can see the rash.

54. What is a "potential" side effect?

If you read about your medication in the *Physicians' Desk Reference* (PDR) or on the fact sheet provided by your pharmacist, you will be confronted with a long list of frightening side effects. These are problems that the drug has the potential to cause. It is your doctor's responsibility to be aware of these, which is why they are listed in the PDR, a thick reference book written for physicians. You may develop one or more of these complications, but probably will not develop any of them. They are *possible* side effects, not *probable* ones.

55. After I get out of bed and take my first dose of medication, I always get dizzy and see double. By late morning, the symptoms go away. What can I do?

Dizziness and double vision are common symptoms of drug toxicity. You have identified exactly when they occur, which will help your doctor fix the problem.

The obvious first choice is to lower the morning dosage; however, this may not be possible if you need the large dose to control your seizures. In that case, try spreading out the pills. Instead of two pills when you wake up, take one, followed by the second pill at 10:00 A.M. In this manner, you will take the same daily amount but will avoid toxic side effects caused by a high blood level.

56. I've gained so much weight since I started my new medication! Why did that happen?

Up to half the patients taking divalproex sodium (Depakote®) gain weight, sometimes large amounts. The drug causes increased appetite, which results in increased weight. Consistent dieting will correct the problem. If the weight gain is severe, the drug may need to be changed. Gabapentin (Neurontin®) and carbamazepine (Tegretol®) can also cause weight gain. [Certain newer antiepileptic drugs, such as felbamate (Felbatol®), topiramate (Topamax®), and zonisamide (Zongegran®), tend to cause weight loss.]

57. My doctor wanted to switch me from one medication to another. But after the first dose I was too dizzy to stand up. What happened?

Replacing one drug with another can be difficult. Frequently, undesirable interactions occur between drugs. For example, when phenytoin (Dilantin®) is added to divalproex sodium (Depakote®), the effective phenytoin level can become too high. The same dose of phenytoin without divalproex sodium would not cause symptoms.

When a new drug is added to your regimen, it is often advisable to decrease the dose of the previous medication. Although lowering one drug risks a seizure, it can prevent toxicity from drug interactions.

58. Do I have to live with all these side effects? They're worse than the epilepsy!

They shouldn't be. There are now a large assortment of effective antiepileptic drugs for you and your doctor to try. These medications work by several different biological mechanisms and have different side effect profiles.

One exception is drowsiness. Some of my patients with difficult-to-control seizures complain of a constant tired feeling. When I lower the dose of their medication, they have breakthrough seizures. Drowsiness is the most difficult side effect to get rid of, as it occurs with nearly all of the medications.

59. Someone told me phenobarbital is addicting. Is that true?

Phenobarbital, primidone (Mysoline®), and mephobarbital (Mebaral®) can be habit-forming. However, they can be excellent, low cost medications to control seizures. I use these drugs with very good results in my practice.

Because the body develops physiologic tolerance to these medications, unpleasant withdrawal symptoms can occur if you suddenly stop taking one of these drugs. You may experience a fast heart rate, tremor, or convulsions. In order to prevent these symptoms, always taper these medications slowly before discontinuing them. Do not "run out."

Last week, one of my patients stopped her primidone abruptly and developed status epilepticus. It corrected as soon as we gave her some phenobarbital in the emergency room.

60. Can medications affect my sex life?

Some antiepileptic drugs can cause impotence in men. Decreased libido and impotence are significantly more frequent with phenobarbital and primidone (Mysoline®) than with other antiepileptic drugs.

Although these problems are of a personal nature, your physician cannot help you with them unless you tell him. Women should alert their gynecologists that they are taking antiepileptic medications.

61. My doctor told me he had to do blood tests every year to check for side effects. What are they?

Some patients develop abnormalities due to certain drugs; for example, carbamazepine (Tegretol®) can lower the number of white blood cells and divalproex sodium (Depakote®) can cause a decrease in the number of blood platelets. Rarely, the white blood cell count becomes too low to fight infection and the drug must be discontinued. Low platelets can cause bleeding problems. The dose of divalproex sodium must be adjusted or the drug stopped if the platelet count is too low.

Many antiepileptic drugs cause abnormalities of liver function. These are usually not severe; however, if they are, the medication must be adjusted or discontinued.

By periodically monitoring your blood, these and other abnormalities can be detected and corrected before they cause symptoms.

6. ALTERNATIVE THERAPY

Danny's mother was an actress. Her seizure disorder was well controlled with phenytoin (Dilantin®). She didn't like taking the medication, but since she had been seizure-free for many years, she was reluctant to stop. Her uncle also had seizures.

Danny was only a "C" student in school, but was artistically talented like his mother. He attended a special school for the arts. Danny had a febrile convulsion at age three. A month after his sixteenth birthday, he had five convulsions in a period of three weeks.

Because of the irregular nature of her work, Danny's mother didn't have health insurance and didn't take him to a doctor. She also was a firm believer in alternative therapies and gave him herbal medications, some from her own organic garden. For a few months, the treatments seemed to work. Then Danny had two more convulsions resulting in a trip to the emergency room. The following day, she took him to see me.

His neurologic examination was normal, but his electroencephalogram (EEG) revealed generalized spike and wave at 3–4 cycles per second. It took me a while to convince Danny and his mother that divalproex sodium (Depakote®), despite its potential side effects, would more likely help Danny than backyard herbs.

62. What were some nonscientific treatments for epilepsy?

Hippocrates (460–357 B.C.) wrote the first scientific paper on epilepsy, *On the Sacred Disease*. He recognized that epilepsy was a disease of the brain due to physical causes. Hippocrates recommended that epilepsy be treated "not by magic, but by diet and drugs."

Nonetheless, an impressive number of useless and unpleasant therapies have been inflicted on patients with epilepsy since then. Here are a few examples: eat a raven's egg or a frog's liver; drink gladiator blood and eat his liver; kill a dog and drink its bile; the person who first saw the patient have a convulsion should urinate into his shoe, stir it, and give it to the patient to drink.

In 1954 Herbert Jasper wrote that the scientific advances made by Hughlings Jackson, William Gowers, and others would lead to "hope" and "more rational therapy" for the person with epilepsy. Modern science has enabled us to move beyond these ancient remedies. (If you have to have epilepsy, it is definitely better to have it now than at any time in the past!)

63. Are there any natural treatments for epilepsy?

The first effective anticonvulsant drug, bromide, is a derivative of the naturally occurring element, bromine. Bromide is not often used today because of its side effects and the ready availability of less toxic antiepileptic drugs.

64. Aren't natural treatments healthier?

The fact that a substance is "natural" does not guarantee either its effectiveness or its safety. Arsenic is a naturally occurring metallic element that can cause diarrhea, cramps, anemia, paralysis, and malignant skin tumors. It was used as a poison gas in World War I. These facts, however, did not keep arsenic from being included as one of the main ingredients in a now forgotten antiepileptic concoction prescribed in the 1930s.

65. Can I control seizures with vitamins?

One type of epilepsy is caused by a deficiency of pyridoxine (vitamin B6). This seizure disorder is rare and usually diagnosed in infancy. Unfortunately, pyridoxine is not useful in treating other forms of epilepsy.

Taking megavitamins has not been shown to help control seizures. Too much of certain vitamins can be harmful.

Very low levels of magnesium and calcium can trigger seizures, but these conditions are infrequent. Patients without a deficiency of these two minerals are unlikely to achieve better seizure control by taking either calcium or magnesium supplements.

66. What about herbal medicines?

No herbs, oils, or potions have been proven to help control seizures. On the other hand, some traditional medicines may have a scientific basis for seizure control.

Herbal medicine has been used in China for over 2,000 years. Qingyangshen is a traditional Chinese medicine that may have antiepileptic properties. Laboratory experiments have shown that a combination of phenytoin and

Qingyangshen can affect gene expression in the brain and reduce seizures in epileptic rats.

A Japanese epilepsy drug, Shosaiko-to-go-keishi-ka-shakuyaku-to, an extract of nine herbs, consists of many known and unknown substances. This preparation has been reported to control seizures in patients. In the laboratory, it can inhibit convulsions in a type of epilepsy-prone mouse.

Both herbal medicines are in the early stages of scientific testing. Where they fit into the modern treatment of epilepsy remains unclear.

67. Why not use herbal medication? Can it do any harm?

There are four significant problems with herbal and other alternative therapies:

+ Despite many promotional claims by manufacturers and others, these drugs have not been proved to work. When a medication has been approved by the Food and Drug Administration (FDA), it has been extensively tested in animals and human beings, at a cost of many millions of dollars. The manufacturer must produce a product with known and consistent ingredients, a profile of expected side effects, specific indications for use, and expected benefits. Herbal remedies available at the health food store are not submitted to this rigorous testing or these strict manufacturing standards. They may be helpful, useless, or dangerous.
+ Herbal medications may have harmful side effects. An example is the Chinese herb "ma huang" ("Herbal Ecstasy"), purported to produce a feeling that "all is right and good with the world." Recent evaluation of this natural therapy by the FDA suggests caution; this drug can cause heart attacks and seizures.
+ Another limitation of traditional medications is that the ingredients are not labeled. Patients may be allergic to the contents and not know it.
+ Perhaps the most persuasive argument against alternative medications is that they can prevent someone from taking a known, effective medication. Based on Danny's strong family history of epilepsy, his normal neurologic examination, and the epileptic pattern on his electroencephalogram, I diagnosed a genetic epilepsy likely to respond to divalproex sodium. His mother's belief in herbal medicine resulted in his having more seizures than necessary. Had he come to me sooner, we could have controlled his seizures and spared him a frightening and expensive trip to the emergency room.

It is likely that additional useful prescription drugs will result from naturally occurring plants and animals. Nature's gardens have already produced drugs for pain control, muscle cramps, congestive heart failure, high blood pressure, and leukemia. Pharmaceutical companies are not blind to the value of naturally occurring medicines. Approximately 25 percent of all prescriptions contain at least one active ingredient from plants.

As yet undiscovered species exist in the oceans and rain forests which may also prove to have therapeutic potential. New research efforts are currently directed toward these promising "alternative therapies."

68. What about biofeedback?

Biofeedback is a group of techniques in which people attempt to consciously control involuntary body functions, such as heart rate, blood pressure, or brain waves. A heart monitor or brain wave machine, for example, provides instant "biofeedback" of the results.

There are reports of seizure control with biofeedback. In one study, patients practiced meditation for 20 minutes each day for a year. They experienced significant brain wave changes as well as a decrease in the duration and frequency of their seizures.

Biofeedback is rarely used in the treatment of epilepsy and has not been well studied. It appears to help some people and has no known side effects. A trial of biofeedback should be considered by highly motivated patients.

69. What about acupuncture?

Acupuncture has been used in both canine and human epilepsy. Acupressure has also been tried to control seizures. There is one report from Anhui Province in China of prompt control of status epilepticus with acupuncture.

The Food and Drug Administration (FDA) recently reclassified acupuncture needles from Class III to Class II devices. This new category removes the "investigational use" labeling requirement and may facilitate increased use of this procedure. It is hoped that more research will be performed as well.

70. Can't I control epilepsy with diet?

There is one specific diet that can be successful in controlling seizures. This is the ketogenic diet, most often prescribed for children. (See Chapter 11.)

71. Can any lifestyle changes help control seizures?

John had a brain tumor removed from his left temporal lobe five years ago. He had no seizures for the first six months after surgery, but then they returned. About once every two weeks, he would have a convulsion. Despite several new medications, he continued to have breakthrough seizures.

I admitted John to the hospital to take a closer look at his seizures on our electroencephalograph and video monitoring equipment (EEG/CCTV). Despite sleep deprivation and withdrawal of his medications, John did not have a single seizure in 17 days of inpatient monitoring.

After repeated interviews about his habits, John finally admitted to the neuropsychologist that he tended to drink "a few beers" every two weeks. It was at this time he had his seizures.

Many patients can drink alcohol without endangering their seizure control, but others cannot. Modification of alcohol intake, including beer, can make a difference in seizure control.

Caffeine stimulates the brain and is an ingredient in coffee, tea, and many soft drinks. Most patients tolerate these beverages without difficulty, but excessive amounts of caffeine can lower the seizure threshold. If you drink more than a few cups of coffee or cans of soda a day, consider cutting back or switching to a decaffeinated brand. This may help with seizure control.

The other important lifestyle factor in seizure control is adequate rest. Whether it is teenagers staying up late to study (or party), pregnant women who cannot sleep, or busy executives with pressing deadlines, seizures can result from sleep deprivation. For many people, a good night's sleep can prevent a seizure from occurring the following day.

72. What about exercise?

Exercise provokes seizures in some patients. However, this is uncommon. The potential benefits of physical fitness, improved mood, and increased socialization outweigh a risk of seizures in most patients. A child or adult should not be discouraged from exercising unless this activity clearly precipitates seizures. Regular exercise may actually improve seizure control.

73. Are there any modern alternative treatments for epilepsy?

A device called the "vagal stimulator" received FDA approval in 1997. (See Chapter 14.) Similar to a cardiac pacemaker, this device sends an electric shock to the vagus nerve in the neck at regular intervals. The vagus nerve transmits the electrical signal to the brain.

In some patients, this pulsed electrical stimulation results in decreased seizure frequency. Several of my patients, while in a research study, have tried it with some improvement. You can get more information about the vagal stimulator from a comprehensive epilepsy center near you and at www.cyberonics.com.

7. BRAIN SURGERY?

The "scary feelings" began when he was ten years old. Sometimes confusion followed these strange sensations. A neurologist determined that Barry had epileptic auras and partial complex seizures.

At first, seizures occurred only once or twice a year. His "scary feeling" usually lasted about 30 seconds, allowing him to drive. But at age 26, a seizure occurred without an aura and Barry had a bad car accident. Luckily, he was not seriously injured. Frightened of what might have happened, Barry gave up his driver's license.

Over the next few years, Barry's seizures increased. He relied on his family, neighbors, and coworkers to get him to and from work. He felt limited as a father because he couldn't drive his son anywhere.

Barry worked hard to get his seizures under control. He took his medication regularly, didn't drink alcohol, got enough sleep, and tried to learn more about epilepsy. At a lecture I gave to an epilepsy support group, he raised his hand and asked if I could help him. We decided to work together.

After trying most of the traditional antiepileptic medications, Barry participated in an investigational drug trial. His seizures improved 30 percent, but it was not enough to allow him to drive. He was afraid of an operation on his brain, but it was his only chance to become seizure-free. Three years ago, Barry had a left temporal lobectomy. Now, at age 41, he's driving a Jaguar.

74. What is epilepsy surgery?

There are several types of surgical operations designed to eliminate seizures. The most common one is anterior temporal lobectomy, in which the front part of the temporal lobe is removed.

Less commonly performed types of epilepsy surgery are corpus callosotomy and hemispherectomy.

75. Can epilepsy surgery be done in children?

Yes. Depending on the type of seizure and epilepsy syndrome, epilepsy surgery can be successfully performed in both children and adults. The youngest patient at our center to have a temporal lobectomy was seven years old. She is now seizure-free.

76. What is a callosotomy?

The two hemispheres of the brain are connected by white matter called the corpus callosum. In a corpus callosotomy, this structure is cut, decreasing the electrical communication between the two halves of the brain. In children with drop attacks, this operation can decrease the sudden falls.

Severing the corpus callosum can help control convulsions in patients who have multiple seizure foci and cannot have a temporal lobectomy.

77. What is a hemispherectomy?

In some people, one hemisphere of the brain has been severely damaged and causes seizures. This operation removes or disconnects that part. Seizures, intellectual function, and social behavior can be surprisingly improved.

78. Is epilepsy surgery new?

No. Wilder Penfield, a famous American neurosurgeon who founded and designed the Montreal Neurological Institute, pioneered this surgery over 50 years ago. By 1954 he had performed over 750 operations. With improved physician training and technology, the surgery has become standardized and refined. As of 1990, over 8000 operations have been done in 118 epilepsy centers worldwide.

79. Will I still have to take medication after the operation?

Most patients require antiepileptic medication in addition to epilepsy surgery to remain seizure-free. Often, the number of drugs and their dosages can be reduced. Some patients will not require any medication.

80. Who performs epilepsy surgery?

After a thorough evaluation by the epilepsy team, a neurosurgeon performs the operation with the assistance of an electrophysiologist, a brain wave specialist.

81. Who is on the "epilepsy team?"

At our comprehensive epilepsy center, the team consists of an epilepsy coordinator, electroencephalograph technologists, a social worker, neuroscience nurses, neuropsychologists, neuropsychiatrists, neurologists, electrophysiologists, and neurosurgeons.

82. Who is a "surgical candidate?"

Candidates for surgery are patients whose seizures significantly decrease quality of life, despite adequate trials of medication.

83. Won't surgery result in a scar on my brain that could cause more seizures?

No. Epilepsy surgery does not cause this problem. We have never had a patient develop a new epilepsy focus as a result of seizure surgery.

84. How can I still be all right after having part of my brain removed?

Most people are understandably reluctant to lose any part of their body, particularly their brain. But epilepsy surgery removes damaged brain. Many people note no loss of function after surgery. (Barry is still working at his accounting job across the street from my office.) Some people even have intellectual improvement, because the damaged part is no longer interfering with normal brain function.

85. Can the surgery make my seizures worse?

No.

86. What is the chance I'll be seizure-free?

This varies for each patient, and you must discuss the expected outcome with your neurologist. Overall, temporal lobectomy eliminates seizures in about 50 percent of patients and at least another 25 percent are significantly improved. Certain patients with a well-defined seizure focus have a 90 percent chance of becoming seizure-free.

87. What testing must be done before the operation?

Patients are admitted to the epilepsy monitoring unit for video/electroencephalograph (CCTV/EEG) localization of their seizure focus. Additionally, they require magnetic resonance imaging (MRI), a neuropsychological evaluation, and a Wada test.

Some centers obtain positron emission tomography (PET) and single photon emission computed tomography (SPECT) scans as well. One or more admissions to the hospital may be required, usually for a total of one to three weeks.

88. Can someone stay with me while I'm being monitored?

In our center, large chairs that convert into beds at night are provided in patient rooms. Family members and close friends become part of the epilepsy team. They are often the first to recognize a seizure when it begins and can notify the nursing staff.

89. What happens in an epilepsy monitoring unit?

Most epilepsy surgery is based on the principle that a single focus of epileptic activity causes the seizures. The purpose of monitoring is to locate that focus so that it can be surgically removed.

Initially, electrodes are pasted to your scalp. Tiny wires, called sphenoidal electrodes, may also be placed under the skin in your cheeks.

If the seizure focus cannot be determined with scalp and sphenoidal electrodes, a surgical procedure to place sterile electrodes inside your skull may be needed. Depending on the situation, the neurosurgeon will place either depth or grid electrodes.

90. Why do I have to see a neuropsychologist? I'm not crazy!

Living with epilepsy produces stress. Being cured of epilepsy by an operation can also be stressful. A neuropsychologist helps patients understand and cope with the many psychosocial issues of epilepsy.

Additionally, a neuropsychologist is trained to evaluate brain function. Extensive testing before the operation helps determine the site of the epileptic focus, as well as the chances of successful surgery. Postoperative testing evaluates whether any changes in thinking, memory, or language have occurred.

All of my presurgical patients are interviewed by our neuropsychologist.

91. What is a Wada test?

A test in which a sedative is injected first into one side of the brain, then the other. This is done in the x-ray department by a neuroradiologist.

The Wada test is done for two reasons. The first is to determine whether speech is located in the right or left temporal lobe. The neurosurgeon needs this information in order to work around the speech center during the operation.

The second purpose is to evaluate memory function. Because part of the memory center is removed during a temporal lobectomy, it is important to make sure the patient will not have noticeable memory loss after the operation. The Wada test determines whether the other temporal lobe works well enough to do the job alone. If the memory centers in both temporal lobes are damaged, the patient may not be able to have surgery.

92. What are depth electrodes?

Successful epileptic surgery requires precise localization of the region in the brain in which the seizures begin. Sometimes the epileptic focus cannot be found using electrodes pasted on the scalp. One option is to insert depth electrodes inside the brain, providing a much better chance of finding the epileptic focus.

93. What is a grid?

A grid is a delicate array of electrodes placed on the surface of the brain by a neurosurgeon. Grids can be useful to localize the seizure focus when it is on the surface of the brain, the cerebral cortex. They are also used for speech mapping.

94. What is speech mapping?

In some patients, the epileptic focus is near the brain's speech center. If so, sometimes an electrophysiologist performs electrical stimulation of the brain to identify the exact location of the speech center. This map helps the neurosurgeon remove all of the epileptic tissue and preserve language function.

95. Will I be awake during the surgery?

Some neurosurgeons prefer to operate on the patient while awake so that speech and other neurologic function can be assessed. Local anesthesia is given and there is no pain. In our center, brain mapping is performed several days before surgery with the patient awake. The actual operation is done with the patient asleep.

96. How long does the surgery take?

A temporal lobectomy typically takes from four to six hours. After surgery, the patient goes to the intensive care unit for a day or two, then to a regular hospital room.

97. How long is the postoperative recovery period?

Most patients leave the hospital after a week. They are back to work in one to three months.

98. What kind of complications can I expect?

Significant medical complications are rare. At our center, two patients had strokes from which they made a near 100 percent recovery. Other problems can occur, such as language or memory difficulties. Some patients have psychological complications, experiencing changes in personality or difficulty adjusting to life with few or no seizures.

Part of the purpose of the extensive presurgical evaluation is to limit the possibility of medical or psychological side effects.

99. How much does epilepsy surgery cost?

In addition to the expense of the surgery itself, anesthesia, operating room, and physician charges, there is the cost of the diagnostic evaluation including hospitalization, epilepsy monitoring, magnetic resonance imaging (MRI), positron emission tomography (PET), single photon emission computed tomography (SPECT), and a neuropsychological evaluation. Depending on the complexity of your case, costs range from $25,000 to $100,000.

100. Will my insurance cover it?

The extent of coverage varies with your individual policy. Speak with the epilepsy coordinator and your insurance representative before beginning the surgery evaluation to answer this question.

101. I want to get rid of my seizures. Can I have epilepsy surgery?

I do not encourage any of my patients to have surgery until they have tried at least three or four medications and worked closely for at least two years with an epilepsy specialist. Additionally, you must be highly motivated.

An epilepsy surgery evaluation typically takes months of time and effort and is expensive. After all the information is obtained, our epilepsy team reviews the patient's history, neurologic examination, neuropsychological results, electroencephalographs (EEGs), monitoring results, and neuroimaging. After a thorough discussion of the findings, we determine the likelihood of benefit from seizure surgery.

At an office visit, I explain the team's recommendations. Then it is up to each patient to decide whether the time, trouble, risks, and expense are worth a chance at seizure control.

8. CAN I DRIVE?

Sam is fifteen years old and has partial complex seizures. He also has diabetes and takes insulin. Two years ago, he went for thirteen months seizure-free, but then the seizures returned. Now he has them one to three times a month. He has tried multiple antiepileptic medications without improvement. Sometimes Sam loses consciousness and it's not clear whether he took too much insulin or had an epileptic seizure. He recently enrolled in a research study with the hope of getting satisfactory seizure control using a new protocol drug.

At his high school, Sam began classroom driver's education classes with the rest of his friends. He asked me when he would be able to start driving lessons in a car. When he learned he had to be seizure-free for a year, he burst out crying. His father asked me when Sam would outgrow his seizures.

102. Why can't Sam learn to drive?

There are two good reasons. The first is that his seizures remain uncontrolled. It is important to note that he experiences partial complex seizures, a type of seizure in which consciousness is altered. With each seizure, Sam becomes confused for several minutes. Clearly, anyone with uncontrolled partial complex seizures should not be driving a moving vehicle.

The second reason is that Sam is having frequent insulin reactions and loses consciousness. He should not be driving a car until he learns to better regulate his diabetes, which will come with experience and more maturity.

103. Can anyone with seizures drive?

Each state has different rules administered by the Department of Motor Vehicles that address this question (see Appendix E). All regulations are attempts to balance the need for the individual to drive against the risk of harm to the driver, his passengers, and anyone else on the road should a seizure occur.

104. Wouldn't it be safe for Sam to drive when he grows out of his seizures?

Yes. Unfortunately, Sam's magnetic resonance imaging (MRI) scan shows left temporal lobe atrophy, an abnormality that will not go away. He does not have a benign childhood epilepsy, such as absence seizures, which he would probably outgrow. I have explained to Sam and his father many times that his type of epilepsy is likely to be lifelong. Although I encourage both of them to be optimistic, and I work very hard with Sam to control his seizures, it is counterproductive to base his future plans on wishful thinking.

105. Will Sam be able to drive if he goes a year seizure-free?

Even though legally he would be able to drive after one year, given Sam's history of recurrent seizures, I would personally like to see him seizure-free a little longer before he gets behind the wheel. I would also like to be confident that he has his diabetes under better control.

106. What about people who only have seizures in their sleep?

A small percentage of patients with epilepsy never have a seizure while awake. They may have one in the daytime while taking a nap, but otherwise only at night in their sleep. (The reason for this is unclear.) These patients may qualify for an exception from the seizure-free period required by their state.

107. What about patients with other seizure types? Can they drive?

Yes. I have one patient who has a seizure every month, yet he is able to drive. He describes a warning in his head. This allows him to prepare for the rest of the seizure. Then his right arm feels as if it is blown up like a balloon, and it moves up and down. Afterwards it feels numb. Although inconvenient, these seizures do not cause any alteration of consciousness and do not significantly interfere with his driving.

Many patients with partial simple seizures that cause minimal symptoms, such as a twitch in the cheek or a tingling in an arm or leg, are able to drive. Generalized seizures, of course, are not compatible with driving.

108. Are there any other circumstances in which a patient with uncontrolled seizures can drive?

Yes. Some patients have prolonged auras. They can sense a seizure coming, either by a "funny feeling," a strong odor, or other warning. If the aura is long enough, they will have time to drive a car to the side of the road. The Department of Motor Vehicles may allow exceptions for these patients.

109. What if my seizures are not controlled and I need to drive to work?

In the United States, public transportation is often lacking, and driving can be essential to function. Unfortunately, needing to drive does not give one the privilege to do so. I have many patients who ride with others. One of my patients, now seizure-free after surgery, shuttles two epilepsy patients from her hometown to their regular visits with me.

You may find some solutions to transportation problems by talking with other people who have epilepsy at local support group meetings or by contacting your Epilepsy Foundation state affiliate.

110. Will my doctor report me if I keep having seizures and continue to drive?

In most states, it is not the physician's legal obligation to notify the Department of Motor Vehicles when patients are having seizures. However, your physician may do this if it appears that you are driving and putting yourself and others at unacceptable risk. Remember, your doctor's primary role is to help you manage your seizures and live as healthy and productive a life as possible.

111. How can I convince my doctor to let me drive?

It is not your doctor you have to persuade. It is the Department of Motor Vehicles; they make the rules. To get a driver's license, make your best effort to work with your doctor to eliminate your seizures. That means taking medication as directed, filling in your seizure calendar, keeping appointments, and being willing to consider sophisticated therapy, such as a protocol drug trial or epilepsy surgery.

If you think you have been unjustly denied a driver's license, ask your doctor for his opinion. If he agrees, consider appealing the decision. Most states permit an appeal.

Whether you can drive or not is a safety issue, a decision that boils down to common sense.

9. SEIZURES AND WORK

Treatment with phenytoin (Dilantin®) and carbamazepine (Tegretol®) didn't stop Bob's seizures. After several years of trial and error, we finally succeeded with a combination of divalproex sodium (Depakote®), gabapentin (Neurontin®), and acetazolamide (Diamox®). Bob also made lifestyle changes (gave up drugs and alcohol) and improved his compliance with medication.

For the past year, Bob has been seizure-free and gainfully employed. Trained as an aircraft engineer, he repairs Teflon strips on propeller blades using chemicals, adhesives, and glues.

Last month I received a letter from his employer noting that Bob had "poor memory for details, increased scrap rate, difficulty following instructions, and multiple mistakes." The employer asked for my advice.

112. Can people with epilepsy work?

A large number of people with epilepsy hold successful careers and work steady jobs. On the other hand, many cannot work. A chart review of 306 of my patients with well-documented epilepsy revealed that 18 percent of them received disability compensation. Unemployment is approximately twice the national average.

113. Why can't people with epilepsy work?

The most frequent problem I see is that seizures interfere with the job. One of my patients worked for the local utility company, maintaining power lines. He pruned trees with a chain saw while standing in a bucket supported two stories above the street by a crane. When he developed epilepsy, it was impractical for him to continue working at this dangerous job.

Many of my patients work in textile mills here in North Carolina. When they develop seizures or their seizures become uncontrolled, it becomes unsafe to continue working with dangerous machinery.

Certain jobs require driving: chauffeuring a taxi or bus, making deliveries, or regional sales. These are all impossible professions for people with uncontrolled seizures.

114. Do people with epilepsy take more sick days than other people?

No. There is no significant difference in days off due to illness. However, patients with epilepsy do use employee health facilities more often.

115. I know someone with epilepsy who doesn't have seizures any more, but she still can't get a job. Why is that?

In some cases, other disabilities associated with epilepsy limit employment.

In children with epilepsy, approximately 9 percent have mental retardation. This additional problem limits their educability and job opportunities in the future.

One of my patients didn't develop epilepsy until he was 20 years old, but he had never worked. He said it was because of his birth defect, a type of cerebral palsy. He has slurred speech and a mild paralysis of his right side with a clumsy right hand.

Sometimes, as in Bob's case, side effects from medication interfere with job performance.

It is also possible that discrimination because of epilepsy can limit job opportunities.

116. How can I keep discrimination from preventing me from getting a job?

Discrimination in employment is outlawed by the Americans with Disabilities Act of 1990, Public Law 101-336. This law supplements the Rehabilitation Act of 1973, which prohibits discrimination by federal contractors, federal agencies, or recipients of federal financial assistance. These laws prevent discrimination in employment on the basis of prejudice and ignorance.

The American with Disabilities Act applies to private businesses with more than 15 employees. Just as it is illegal to discriminate on the basis of race or sex, this law makes it illegal to discriminate on the basis of epilepsy. However, the person applying for the job must be willing and able to do the job.

117. What if they ask for a drug test? Do I have to take it?

Yes. Drug tests are designed to screen for drug abuse and can be required before or after a job offer is given. However, the presence of epilepsy drugs in your result cannot be used to disqualify you for the job.

118. What about a medical examination?

An employer is not permitted to ask health-related questions during an interview or on a job application. A medical history and examination can only be required after a job offer is made. It is illegal for an employer to use the fact that you have epilepsy to disqualify you.

119. How does the Americans with Disabilities Act protect me?

Another feature of the Americans with Disabilities Act is the "reasonable accommodation" provision. This language requires the employer to make changes in the work environment or job description if the applicant can otherwise fulfill all the "essential functions" of employment.

My patient Karen was in her early forties and had a successful banking job. She worked in administration, where her monthly partial complex seizures were not a major problem. She usually would have a brief warning and sit down at her desk or go to the ladies room until the seizure was over. She did her work well and was advancing in management.

Last year, the bank acquired its first out of town branch office, which required an inspection every three months. Branch supervision was part of Karen's responsibility. She had never had a problem with this before, as she could take a cab to all the local branches. In order to inspect this new rural acquisition, she would have to take a short flight and then rent a car. Because of her seizures, traveling presented a problem.

Although it was her responsibility, this particular branch inspection could be performed by one of her colleagues. It was also a very small part of her job, not an "essential function." Consequently, when Karen asked her boss to relieve her of this obligation, the only aspect of her job she could not do, she was protected by the Americans with Disabilities Act. It was possible for her boss to make a "reasonable accommodation" by assigning this trip to someone else and letting Karen continue doing her good work at the home office.

120. Does the Americans with Disabilities Act keep me from getting fired?

Jack worked at a nature museum. Initially, his seizures were controlled, but as he got older his epilepsy became more severe. Despite increasing doses of medication, he began having seizures at work and would become confused and wander off.

Jack's primary job was feeding the animals and cleaning their cages. Some of the animals, such as raccoons and foxes, were potentially dangerous. One day, while bringing breakfast to a valuable arctic fox, he had a seizure and left the cage open. When his mind cleared and he realized what had happened, he searched all over the museum, but he couldn't find the fox.

The next day, the animal was found dead on a nearby highway. Jack was fired when the details of the incident became clear to his employer.

Jack was furious over losing his job and contacted a lawyer. He said he wanted to sue because of discrimination. The attorney advised Jack that the law did not protect him in this case. He was not being discriminated against because he had epilepsy. He was let go because his uncontrolled seizures did not allow him to do his job properly or safely.

121. Who should I contact if I have a concern about discrimination?

Call your state affiliate or the national office of the Epilepsy Foundation (EF). They will be able to provide you with more information and direct you to the proper legal resources. An informative booklet, *The Americans with Disabilities Act, A Guide to Provisions Affecting Persons with Seizure Disorders*, is also available from the EF.

122. Who at work should I tell?

If it is likely that you will have a seizure at work, you should inform your supervisor and close coworkers. Otherwise, after your first seizure on the job, you will probably get whisked off to the emergency room. Your coworkers will be best prepared to help you if they are forewarned.

When you discuss your epilepsy, you will have an opportunity to educate your coworkers about appropriate first aid. You can also give them guidelines regarding when to call an ambulance. If your supervisor wants more information, you can suggest that he call your doctor, a local epilepsy center, or the EF.

123. Should I wear a Medic Alert bracelet?

This is a personal decision. Some people are private about their seizures. Others, particularly those with frequent seizures, have learned that communication about their disorder can benefit them. For example, if a police officer finds you confused in a parking lot late Saturday night, he is likely to consider epilepsy rather than alcohol intoxication when he sees a Medic Alert bracelet.

Some patients prefer to wear a Medic Alert necklace, as this is more discreet but would be found by health professionals or others in an emergency. Ask your doctor for his opinion.

124. What if I can't find a job?

Finding the right job is difficult for everyone. Frequent seizures increase the likelihood of unemployment. Work with your doctor to control your seizures.

If you continue to have difficulty finding a job, look to others who may be able to help you. If you are in school, career counselors are available. If you have finished school, ask your doctor for a referral to a social worker or vocational rehabilitation. Ask about a referral to JobTech.

125. What is JobTech?

JobTech is a new employment program developed by the Epilepsy Foundation and sponsored by the US Department of Labor and the US Social Security Administration. JobTech helps people with epilepsy find jobs in the technology-based customer service field.

JobTech had its first program year in 2000-1 and is currently administered by four epilepsy affiliates; Camden, NJ, Kansas City, MO, Mobile, AL, and Rockford, IL (see Appendix C). Other local affiliates also offer assistance with job finding.

(JobTech replaces a prior program, Training Applicants for Placement Success [TAPs], which was funded by the US Department of Labor and had been in operation since 1976.)

126. My seizures are perfectly controlled. Are there any jobs I still can't qualify for?

The federal Department of Transportation prohibits anyone with a history of seizures from obtaining a federal commercial driver's license. Similarly, the

Federal Aviation Administration disqualifies anyone with a history of epilepsy from becoming a commercial pilot.

There are no other legal restrictions that prevent people with controlled seizures from working.

127. What about the armed forces?

Enlistment in one of the branches of the armed forces is possible if you are seizure-free without medications for at least five years.

128. What happened to Bob? Did his work performance improve?

I made sure his drug levels weren't toxic, and Bob tried without success to boost the quality of his work. I wrote a letter on his behalf, but Bob lost his job. Even though he wasn't having seizures, he was not able to meet the required standards of his position. Now he works for another company as a fluid hydraulics mechanic and seems to be doing fine.

10. Women and Epilepsy

Jill was 22 years old and four months pregnant when we met at the obstetrics clinic two years ago. It was the first time she had seen a neurologist since she was a teenager. Even though she had not had a seizure in years, she was still taking two epilepsy medications. Her pregnancy was going well and she was reluctant to decrease her medications for fear of a seizure. After she delivered (luckily, a healthy baby), I ordered a sleep-deprived electroencephalogram (EEG) and magnetic resonance imaging (MRI) scan. Since both studies were normal, we decided to decrease her to one medication with the intention of stopping it eventually if she continued seizure-free.

Although Jill insisted she had no plans for another baby, she reluctantly agreed to take prenatal vitamins and folate. She had her drug level checked regularly and we kept it in the low therapeutic range. Last month she appeared in the obstetrics clinic again, embarrassed but with a smile on her face. She was pregnant again! We both felt reassured that we had done everything we could to ensure a healthy baby.

129. Why do I have seizures only around the time of my period?

A few women have seizures related to their monthly cycle. This is called catamenial epilepsy. Hormonal changes at this time lower the seizure threshold. Use your seizure calendar to see whether your seizures only occur with your period. If you have catamenial epilepsy, your doctor may want to prescribe acetazolamide (Diamox®), which may help control this type of seizure.

130. Will taking birth control pills cause me to have more seizures?

Usually birth control pills will not affect seizure frequency (but see the next question).

131. Will the birth control pill reduce the efficacy my epilepsy medication?

No, but some medications, including carbamazepine (Tegretol®), oxcarbazepine (Trileptal®), phenobarbital, phenytoin (Dilantin®), primidone (Mysoline®), and topiramate (Topamax®) can increase the metabolism of the birth control pill and render it less effective. If you are taking one of these medications, you must consult your obstetrician to see if you need a stronger dosage of the birth control pill or a different form of contraception.

Divalproex sodium (Depakote®), gabapentin (Neurontin®), lamotrigine (Lamictal®), levetiracetam (Keppra®), and zonisamide (Zonegran®) do not affect the birth control pill.

132. What about levonorgestrel implants (Norplant®) or medroxyprogesterone (Depo-Provera®)?

The same cautions given for the birth control pill apply. One of my patients became pregnant while taking carbamazepine (Tegretol®) and using the levonorgestrel implant. She wasn't ready for another child and the pregnancy caused a great deal of stress.

133. What is the best medication for treating seizures in pregnancy?

Although you may hear differently, it is now generally agreed that the best choice of epilepsy medication in pregnancy is the drug that eliminates the most seizures with the fewest side effects. No medication has proved "safer" than any other.

134. How will pregnancy affect my seizure frequency?

Seizure frequency may increase during pregnancy. Part of the reason for this increase is that many women stop their epilepsy medications. This is usually not the best thing to do.

Seizures may also occur because pregnancy can cause poor absorption of medication and an increase in drug metabolism, both of which result in lower drug levels. In order to have the best control of seizures during pregnancy, it is essential to visit both your obstetrician and neurologist regularly. Because of the dramatic changes in your body, you will need to have drug levels measured more frequently. Your dosage may need to be increased, particularly during the third trimester, and then decreased promptly after delivery.

Another cause of increased seizures is lack of sleep. To avoid seizures, you must make a special effort to get enough rest.

135. Should I discontinue my epilepsy medications if I become pregnant?

Although medications can cause birth defects, they usually do not. The risk of birth defects in children to women with epilepsy is about 6 percent. That means there is a 94 percent chance there will be no birth defects.

The most serious birth defects occur early in pregnancy, before you even know you're pregnant. That is why stopping your medication will probably increase your seizures and not help your baby very much.

You should not discontinue medication until you have consulted your physician. The risk of harm to you and your baby is probably greater if you have a convulsion than the risk to your baby from medication. If you are taking antiepileptic medication, you may receive educational materials and participate in the AED Pregnancy Registry by calling 1-888-233-2334.

136. Is there a way to check for birth defects?

Yes. One blood test is called "alpha-fetoprotein," which you should get at approximately 18 weeks, particularly if you are taking carbamazepine (Tegretol®) or divalproex sodium (Depakote®). It is also important to get an ultrasound at this time.

137. I am taking three anticonvulsants. Is this worse than taking just one?

Yes. Planning your pregnancy with your doctor is an excellent opportunity to reevaluate your medicines. If your seizures are controlled, perhaps two medications would be sufficient. (Jill was able to do just fine on one.) This would lower the danger to your baby and decrease the likelihood that you will have side effects from the medications. You can work with your neurologist to adjust your medications so that you are taking the least number of drugs at the lowest dosages necessary to control your seizures.

138. What can I do to make sure I have a healthy baby?

Plan your pregnancy! That way you can begin taking prenatal vitamins, make sure you eat nutritious foods, get enough sleep, and avoid alcohol, drugs, and cigarettes.

139. Are there any special vitamins I should take?

Yes. Before you become pregnant, you should take prenatal vitamins. If you are a sexually active woman of childbearing age, you should at the very least take a multivitamin every day, even if you are not planning to become pregnant.

Some doctors also prescribe additional folic acid (1–4 mg), which may help prevent birth defects of the brain and spinal cord.

At about 36–38 weeks, your doctor may also prescribe vitamin K, which can help prevent bleeding in the baby at the time of delivery.

140. Can seizures occur during delivery?

Yes, but only 1 to 2 percent of women with epilepsy have a convulsion during labor and delivery. This is a time of high stress. But seizures can be easily treated in the delivery room with intravenous medication such as diazepam (Valium®) or lorazepam (Ativan®).

141. Can I breast-feed?

Epilepsy medication appears in the breast milk to some degree but usually does not affect the infant. Phenobarbital and primidone (Mysoline®) can cause drowsiness in the baby and poor sucking. If this happens, you will have to bottle-feed. Otherwise, breast-feeding should not be a problem.

142. Will my seizures interfere with taking care of the baby?

If you have frequent partial complex or grand mal seizures, it may be unsafe for you to be the sole caretaker of an infant. There are some things you can do to lower the risks. When changing the baby, for example, do it on the floor rather than on a high table. Do not bathe the baby yourself. Try to find someone to help you with child care so that you do not become overtired.

Some women with frequent seizures cannot safely take care of a baby. You and your doctor should make this important decision together.

11. MY CHILD WITH EPILEPSY

Jessica is a five-year-old girl I saw in the emergency room for her first seizure. She and her grandmother sleep in the same bed. Her grandmother told me that Jessica began "jerking and gasping" at five o'clock in the morning. She was unresponsive and staring, and the jerking lasted about fifteen minutes. Jessica had been coughing a little for the past few days, but had no fever. After the convulsion, her right side seemed weak.

When I examined her, she had a low-grade temperature and slight wheezes in both lungs. Her strength had returned to normal. Jessica's computed axial tomography (CAT) scan was unremarkable. Her electroencephalogram (EEG) revealed large spikes on the left side of her brain.

I was able to reassure her distressed grandmother that Jessica had a benign focal epilepsy of childhood, Rolandic epilepsy, which she would probably outgrow. The seizure had been triggered by her bronchitis. Because the convulsion was so upsetting and prolonged, we decided to treat Jessica with antiepileptic medication until she no longer needed it.

143. Will my child grow out of her seizures?

Your neurologist can help you with prognosis by diagnosing the particular epileptic syndrome. The history, physical examination, brain imagining, and particularly the electroencephalogram (EEG) all help your doctor arrive at an accurate classification of your child's epilepsy.

For example, if your child has Rolandic epilepsy, a benign partial seizure of childhood, she will likely outgrow it during adolescence. On the other hand, if she has Lennox-Gastaut syndrome, she probably will not.

Although epilepsy can rarely be cured, much can be gained by obtaining an accurate diagnosis. This helps guide treatment and molds expectations for the future. (Had Jessica not been evaluated in the emergency room, her grandmother would have worried needlessly that Jessica would suffer seizures all her life.)

144. What is a febrile seizure?

Small children can have convulsions related to a high fever. Febrile seizures are common, occurring in 4 percent of children. When a first seizure occurs with fever, the child should be evaluated by a physician. A respiratory infection or gastroenteritis often causes the elevated temperature. If the seizure is prolonged, anticonvulsants will be needed, the body has to be cooled, and the underlying cause of the fever must be treated. Most doctors do not prescribe daily anticonvulsants after a first febrile seizure. If one child has febrile seizures, the risk of other siblings developing febrile seizures is ~8 percent.

Children outgrow febrile seizures by the age of five or six years. The vast majority do not go on to develop epilepsy. Risk factors for epilepsy are a pre-existing neurologic abnormality, onset of febrile seizures before one year of age, multiple or prolonged febrile seizures, and a family history of epilepsy. If your child has none of these risk factors, the likelihood of epilepsy is only about 1 percent.

145. Why can't they find a cause for the seizure? They told me all her tests are normal!

In more than 50 percent of children with epilepsy, no brain tumor, cyst, malformation, or "scar" explains the occurrence of a seizure. However, an intermittent electrical malfunction in the child's brain is responsible. Although the electroencephalogram (EEG) can be normal between seizures, the abnormal brain waves will usually be seen if a seizure occurs during an EEG.

When all the tests are normal and no cause is found, this is a good sign. These children's seizures tend to be more easily controlled.

146. Do seizures cause brain damage?

Children with absence or petit mal seizures can have many spells without apparent ill effects. After a staring spell, they can pick up where they left off in a conversation. Their electroencephalogram (EEG) returns to normal immediately.

Patients with partial complex or generalized seizures, however, do not return to normal right away. The postictal period immediately after a seizure is characterized by confusion and fatigue. The EEG often slows after a seizure, supporting the concept that the brain has not fully recovered.

We do know that brain injury can occur when seizures last longer than 30 minutes. Two of my adult patients had significant memory loss after episodes of status epilepticus.

Whether brief seizures cause brain injury is unknown. Much research is currently focused on answering this question. Many of my patients with intractable temporal lobe epilepsy complain of memory difficulties. Whether this problem stems from their numerous seizures or the underlying cause of the epilepsy remains unclear.

It does appear prudent to control seizures when possible. Even though medications have potential side effects, they are usually a better choice than recurrent seizures.

147. What is the ketogenic diet?

Diet treatments for epilepsy have been prescribed for epilepsy since the time of Hippocrates. But the only diet proven to help children with epilepsy is the ketogenic diet.

Pioneered over 80 years ago at Johns Hopkins University, the ketogenic diet is low in carbohydrate and protein and extremely high in fat. The diet contains up to five times more fat than protein and carbohydrates combined. It is what most adults would consider a very unhealthy diet. However, because of the calorie restriction, children do not gain excess weight. The fat in the diet causes molecules called ketone bodies to accumulate. For reasons we do not understand, a large number of these in the blood can decrease seizure frequency.

Because of its complexity, the ketogenic diet can only be followed under a physician's supervision with the assistance of a dietitian. The diet begins with a hospital admission for three to five days for fasting and meal preparation training. The diet must be followed exactly. Each food portion is carefully weighed on a scale, and the entire meal must be eaten.

If the diet is going to be effective, seizure frequency decreases within a month. Under the best of circumstances, the child becomes seizure-free. After two years of successful seizure control, the diet can be discontinued without return of seizures. But the diet does not work in every child.

Carrying out this diet requires a strong parental commitment and your child's continuous cooperation. If you are interested, discuss the diet with your pediatric neurologist. You may need to go to a comprehensive epilepsy center to find a dietitian familiar with this program.

If you wish to learn more about the ketogenic diet, an excellent book has been written for parents, dietitians, and physicians which should answer your questions. *The Epilepsy Diet Treatment: An Introduction to the Ketogenic Diet* can be obtained from Demos Medical Publishing, 386 Park Avenue South, New York, N.Y., 10016, (800) 532-8663.

148. Are epilepsy and attention deficit disorder (ADD) related?

Epilepsy affects 1 to 2 percent of children, while ADD affects 3 to 10 percent. Since these disorders are relatively common, some children have both. But there is no connection between the two.

Although deficits in attention can be caused by seizures, epilepsy is rarely the culprit in children with ADD. (Children with epilepsy will be inattentive during their seizures and the postictal period, but the rest of the time their attention is normal.)

Most children with ADD do not have epilepsy. If there is any question about the diagnosis, take your child to see a pediatric neurologist who will take a detailed history, examine your child, and order an electroencephalogram (EEG).

149. Can video games cause seizures?

About 5 percent of people with epilepsy have seizures (called photosensitive epilepsy) in response to flashing lights. Children and adults with this type of seizure disorder need to avoid strobe lights, flickering television screens, and video games.

Sometimes children have their first seizure triggered by a video game, making it appear that the game caused their epilepsy. This is not the case. Children without epilepsy do not have seizures from video games.

Most children with epilepsy are not photosensitive. Before prohibiting your child from playing video games and watching television, ask your neurologist whether flashing lights present a risk.

150. Can my child participate in sports?

One of the dangers of epilepsy is the overprotectiveness it fosters in parents. To develop normally, children need to face many challenges, academic, social, and athletic, among others. To have a full life, they need to test their limits (and probably yours!).

Children with frequent seizures should not swim alone, horseback ride, rock climb, high dive, do gymnastics above the ground on the balance beam and rings, or participate in other sports in which a sudden loss of consciousness could result in serious injury. Baseball, soccer, football, tennis, volleyball, and playground sports are safer. Children with less frequent seizures can participate in most sports. Exercise rarely causes seizures.

There is always the possibility of injury when participating in sports, even for a child without epilepsy. As a parent, you will have to weigh the risk of injury against the risk of depriving your child of an important facet of life. Discuss safety concerns with your child, his teacher, coach, and physician. If your child rides a bicycle, a helmet is a good precaution. While boating, every child should wear a life jacket.

151. I want my child to know he isn't the only one with epilepsy. What can I do?

A local support group where your child can meet other children with seizures may be helpful. The Epilepsy Foundation (EF) sponsors a School Alert program to provide epilepsy education. An educational puppet show, "Kids on the Block," is available for children. Contact the EF to see whether a program can be done in your child's classroom. Knowledge of epilepsy can replace fear and provide a more supportive classroom environment for your child.

There are more than 30 summer camps across the nation for children with epilepsy. Some are free of charge or scholarships may be available through the local affiliate. These camps provide an exposure to sports under supervision as well as an opportunity to interact with peers. (See Appendix F.)

12. Epilepsy and the Elderly

Eleanor had a stroke at age 66, while recovering in the intensive care unit after a difficult heart operation. Her right arm and leg became weak and she had difficulty finding the right words. After a month in a rehabilitation hospital, she regained all of her strength and went home with only a slight hesitancy of speech.

A few months later, while eating breakfast, Eleanor's right arm suddenly began jerking and she slumped over unconscious. A minute or two later, she woke up and found her pancakes in her lap. Her head hurt and she couldn't figure out what had happened. She got her neighbor to drive her to the emergency room. A computed axial tomography (CAT) scan found evidence of her old stroke, but no new problem. Two weeks later, she had another spell. This time she bit her tongue. After another visit to the hospital, a neurologic consultation, and an electroencephalogram (EEG), the doctors told her she had epilepsy.

152. Why do older people develop epilepsy?

Epilepsy is a disorder of neurons in the brain. Whenever these are damaged, seizures can result. New cases of epilepsy tend to occur in young people because of brain injury before and after birth. Inherited seizure disorders also typically manifest themselves before the age of 20. After the age of 65, acquired insults to the brain, such as stroke, brain tumors, and infections cause epilepsy.

153. What is the most common cause of epilepsy in the elderly?

As in Eleanor's case, new seizures in older people are most often caused by stroke.

154. How can you determine the cause?

All patients with new onset seizures, regardless of their age, must see their physician for a complete evaluation. This will consist of a history, physical examination, and usually an electroencephalograph (EEG) and brain scan, such as a computed axial tomography (CAT) or magnetic resonance imaging (MRI).

155. So many older people get Alzheimer's disease. Can it cause epilepsy too?

Yes. Patients with Alzheimer's disease have an increased risk of developing seizures.

156. What are other common causes of seizures in the elderly?

Tumors and infections of the brain can provoke seizures. Collections of blood that put pressure on the brain can also cause seizures.

157. Is epilepsy treatment different in the elderly?

The principles are the same. Treatment begins with identifying the cause. For example, a seizure may be the first warning that a brain tumor is developing. Treatment of the tumor with surgery may eliminate the seizures.

In many cases, there is no surgical cure for the cause of the seizures. Some brain tumors are inoperable, and there is no surgical treatment for the vast majority of strokes. In these situations, effective therapy depends on antiepileptic medications.

158. Which are the best medications to use in older people?

The choice of antiepileptic medication is always complicated, especially in the elderly. The seizure type must first be identified, and your doctor will do this based on the clinical setting, electroencephalogram (EEG), and brain imaging results. Additional factors to consider are the decreased kidney and liver function in many older people, as well as the possibility for drug interactions with commonly used medications such as anticoagulants, calcium channel blockers, quinidine, cimetidine, theophylline, and others.

159. Are drug dosages the same in the elderly?

Typically, less medication is given because of the factors mentioned previously. Lower doses are also preferable because the elderly are more likely to develop drowsiness or confusion from antiepileptic drugs.

160. How do you determine the right dose?

The right dose of medication is the least amount that controls the seizures and causes the fewest and mildest side effects. Accurate communication with your doctor by phone, keeping your seizure calendar, regular doctor visits, and periodic measurement of serum drug levels are dependable ways to make sure you are taking the right dose.

161. How can I avoid drug interactions?

Once your dose is well regulated, it is important to inform your neurologist if one of your other doctors makes any changes in the other medications you take. For example, beginning cimetidine can raise the level of phenytoin, resulting in symptoms of toxicity.

Bring all your medication bottles to each doctor visit. You can write down any medication changes in the personal medical history section in the back of this book.

13. First Aid and Safety Tips

I saw Carol for the first time in the emergency room. She was fumbling with the sheets on the stretcher and appeared confused. She didn't respond when I talked to her. I quickly interviewed her husband and began a neurologic examination.
Suddenly her body stiffened and she began to jerk. Her lips turned blue and she bit her tongue. Blood trickled down her chin onto the pillow. I stood next to her and watched, making sure she didn't hurt herself. Her husband backed into the corner, horrified. The jerking stopped after what seemed like an hour, but was in fact only 90 seconds. Carol took loud, deep breaths. The nurse came in and helped me turn her on her side. I completed my examination, wrote admitting orders, and went to see my next patient.

The following morning I got a call from the hospital administrator. My patient's husband was furious that I had allowed his wife to "have a seizure" and that "the doctor didn't do anything." The administrator demanded an explanation.

162. The patient had a seizure. Why didn't you do anything?

The most important thing to do during a seizure is to prevent patients from injuring themselves. When a patient has a convulsion, remove hard objects such as tables or chairs from their path. Protect the head by putting something soft under it, a pillow or jacket, even just your foot, so that the person's head does not bang on the floor or ground.

When you can, turn the person on his side to prevent saliva from blocking the airway. It is not advisable to stick something into the person's mouth. People can bite their tongue or cheeks during a convulsion. However, because this occurs early in the seizure, you are not likely to prevent it. Trying to force a spoon or stick between clenched teeth also risks breaking a tooth, which the patient may then swallow or inhale. (Do not worry that the person will "swallow his tongue." This does not occur. I have witnessed hundreds of convulsions, and we have not lost a tongue yet!)

When patients have confusional episodes, prevent them from injury. Touch them as little as possible and do not restrain them. If you do, they may resist, and you will have a fight on your hands. Talk softly and be reassuring. Try not to be frightened.

Donna, a large woman on the epilepsy monitoring unit, started walking out of her room during a seizure, trailing her wires behind her. This was potentially dangerous because she was hooked up with depth electrodes in her brain and she was running out of slack. As she approached me in the doorway, I gently turned her 180 degrees. She walked back into the room without missing a step.

Carol was on a stretcher with the guard rails up. She was in no danger of falling. My biggest concern was that she would strike her head, and I watched carefully to see that this did not happen. Her skin color and breathing improved promptly. I examined her movements to see if there was any asymmetry that might point to a seizure focus.

I did not inject her with diazepam (Valium®) for two reasons. First, I would have had to leave the bedside to get it. Second, by the time I was ready, the seizure would have run its course and the diazepam would have just made her sleepy.

I should have explained to her husband what had happened. At the time, I was preoccupied with getting Carol into the hospital and treating her to prevent another seizure. The next day she was fine and went home on medication. Before she left, I gave her and her husband first aid instructions and several pamphlets from the Epilepsy Foundation. I scheduled an appointment for them with the nurse at our comprehensive epilepsy center for additional epilepsy education. (I should probably have asked our hospital administrator to attend as well.)

163. When should I ask for an ambulance?

This is a judgment call. Knowing the patient makes the decision much easier. Jean has light seizures characterized by slight confusion and humming. Her family has learned by experience that whenever her humming lasts longer than a few minutes, she will have a convulsion. In her case, one convulsion leads to another and she develops status epilepticus. When Jean hums, they immediately take her to the emergency room.

One useful guideline for an observer is that the jerking and stiffening of a convulsion should not last more than two minutes. Any longer, and an ambulance should be called. If you can, time the seizure. A convulsion that lasts only a minute can seem a lot longer.

The drowsy phase after a seizure should not last longer than 15 minutes. By this time, patients should be alert enough to answer appropriately or say their names. Ask simple questions that require a specific answer. For example, "what day is it?,", "where are you?,", "does anything hurt you?,", "do you have epilepsy?"

If you do not get a proper answer after 15 minutes, call an ambulance. (A reply of "O.K." is not adequate evidence that the patient has recovered. After a seizure, Terry says "O.K." to every question. If you ask, "are you all right?," he will say "O.K." If you ask, "would you like to fly to the moon?," he will also say "O.K.")

Check to see whether the patient has any injuries. Is there blood? Can the person walk without staggering? Because it is often difficult to know whether someone requires hospitalization, try to get some assistance with this decision. Call a family member or the patient's doctor. Check for a Medic Alert bracelet or necklace.

Most patients with epilepsy have single brief convulsions that do not require hospitalization. After five or ten minutes of postictal confusion, they may be tired, have sore muscles, and complain of a headache, but do not need immediate medical attention. Often they need to rest or go to sleep before resuming their normal activities.

Ask the person what he would like to do after a seizure. Does he want to go to the hospital? Does he want you to call his doctor? Does he need to find a ride? Tell the patient what happened. Be calm and supportive. A person may be embarrassed at having a seizure in public and may have soiled his clothes. Stay with him until he can take care of himself or someone else comes to help.

If it is a first seizure, call an ambulance. The patient should go to the emergency room for a complete evaluation.

164. I live by myself and have convulsions about twice a month. I don't always have a warning. How can I make my home safer?

Years ago, when most homes were heated by open fires, many people with epilepsy sustained burns due to falls into the hearth. Although heating is more modern now, burns from fireplaces, ovens, and hot water are still real problems.

Every home has two particularly dangerous areas, the kitchen and the bathroom. A number of minor modifications can decrease the likelihood of serious accidents:

KITCHEN

The short periods of confusion during and after a complex partial seizure predispose to injury. While cooking, you may place hands or arms on a burner or spill hot food on yourself. In order to avoid this, use oven mitts and cook only on the rear burners.

An electric stove eliminates an open flame and the worry that you might leave the gas on. The safest option is to cook with a microwave. A microwave heats food behind a closed door and shuts off automatically. Microwave cookbooks are available.

To avoid dropping hot food during a seizure, keep a cart in the kitchen that you can wheel to the table.

Tap water can become hot enough to scald. Ask your plumber to install a heat control device in the kitchen faucet to prevent the water from becoming dangerously hot.

Consider carpeting the kitchen floor. Although not as easy to clean, it is much more comfortable to land on.

Whenever possible, use plastic containers rather than glass.

BATHROOM

One of my patients let the hot water run in the tub during a seizure and severely burned both feet. This type of injury can be prevented by installing a temperature control device in the tub and shower heads.

There are many hard surfaces in the bathroom—the sink, the tub, the toilet—that you can't do much about, but you can carpet the floor. Carpet is softer and less slippery than tile.

Do not put a lock on the bathroom door. If you have one, don't use it. It will be difficult for someone to help you after a seizure if they cannot get in.

Learn to take a bath with only a few inches of water in the tub. Use a handheld shower head. If you have frequent seizures, bathe with supervision.

Stairs can be dangerous. If possible, choose a ranch house or one floor apartment rather than a townhouse. If you have stairs, try to arrange your routine to limit how often you must go from floor to floor.

Use more carpet! Avoid shiny hardwood floors.

If you have a fireplace, keep a protective glass screen in front of it.

Irons can get very hot. Buy one that shuts off automatically.

Avoid curling irons. They give a nasty burn.

Another household hazard is cigarettes. To decrease the risk of fire, do not smoke in the house. Better yet, do not smoke! Install smoke alarms in each room.

165. My seizures usually occur early in the morning when I have stayed up late. What can I do?

Some patients know when they are likely to have seizures. Certain circumstances, such as sleep deprivation, missed medication, or time of the month, may herald the onset of a convulsion. An increase in myoclonic jerks may suggest that a seizure will soon follow.

On days when they are at high risk for seizures because of sleep deprivation, I ask my patients to stay in bed a little longer. If they do have a convulsion, it will happen in a soft bed, not running down the stairs to catch a bus. If they have missed medication, they need to make it up. If it is a high risk time of the month, they should avoid potentially dangerous activities such as bicycle riding or boating.

A little prevention can eliminate the need for a lot of first aid.

14. CLINICAL RESEARCH: SHOULD I PARTICIPATE IN A DRUG TRIAL?

Jim is a 35-year-old man I have treated for five years. He has partial complex seizures about 12 times a month. First he notices an aura of a heavy feeling in his tongue, then he will stare, chew, cough, and become confused. Sometimes he falls. He has broken a rib and fractured both great toes due to seizures.

Despite trying five medications, his seizures continued. We studied him in the epilepsy monitoring unit and discovered that the seizures began in at least three separate regions of his brain. Consequently, he was not a surgical candidate. His mother, who still looks after him, asked me whether there was anything else we could try.

Three years ago, I started Jim on a protocol drug. His seizure frequency has slightly reduced, down to eight a month. He and his mother also note that the seizures are briefer and less severe. The only side effect he has from the medication is a tremor.

166. What is a drug trial?

Before a new epilepsy medication can be released on the market, the manufacturer must demonstrate to the Food and Drug Administration (FDA) that the medication is safe and effective. In order to do this, new medications are first tested in animals, then in healthy human volunteers, then in patients with epilepsy. All human testing must be approved by the FDA. Each study design must also be approved by an institutional review board (IRB), composed of health care professionals and lay persons, to ensure that the study meets ethical standards.

167. Why doesn't my doctor prescribe one of the new drugs for me?

An investigational drug can only be given to a patient under the auspices of a clinical trial. It cannot be prescribed until it is approved by the FDA.

A drug study requires a huge commitment of time and energy from each patient as well as the physician and nurses conducting the study. Patients must record each seizure carefully and take every dose of medication exactly as directed. To check on compliance, at each visit a nurse will count all the pills left in the medication bottles. Trips to the doctor are frequent and can be lengthy (often two hours or more).

After the FDA has approved the study, the principal investigator (PI) at each site must attend a conference at which the study goals and limitations are discussed. Then the physician must justify the project to the IRB, keep careful records (typically in triplicate), repeatedly examine patients in great detail, and review hundreds of pages of laboratory data. The site must pass inspection by the pharmaceutical company and prepare for possible examination by the FDA.

Because of the amount of organization, facilities, and time required for a drug study, this type of epilepsy research is performed at medical schools or comprehensive epilepsy centers.

168. What is a drug protocol?

A protocol is a specific plan that spells out exactly how the research will be performed. Each study has its own protocol, which must be followed exactly for the results to have scientific value. For example, the protocol dictates the medication dose patients receive, how often they must come for a check-up, and which type of testing is necessary, such as electroencephalograms, electrocardiograms, blood tests, and urine samples.

Most epilepsy clinical trials are performed at several locations, or sites. By following the protocol, the doctors at each site perform the study exactly the same way.

169. When should I consider a drug study?

For most patients, a drug study should be considered when conventional therapy has failed. Jim had already tried most of the available medications, and he was not a surgical candidate. A clinical trial held the promise of a new drug that might be helpful but would not be available by prescription for years. Additionally, Jim and his mother would get the reassurance of frequent doctor visits and blood monitoring. Another benefit of enrolling in a drug study is the satisfaction of knowing that the results of this clinical research will help other people with epilepsy.

170. How do I know it is safe?

Part of the purpose of a drug study is to determine whether the new medication causes side effects in patients. Consequently, there is no guarantee that the drug is safe.

In order to protect patients, study protocols typically require frequent doctor visits, during which the patient receives a full physical and neurologic examination, as well as blood and urine tests. Patients are encouraged to keep in contact by phone. In this manner, if there is a dangerous side effect, it will be found early. In my experience, serious problems are rare.

There are definite risks to participating in a drug study. However, the risk of not participating is likely to be continued uncontrolled seizures.

171. How much does it cost to participate in a study?

In many instances, the cost of the investigational medication, clinic visits, and laboratory testing is borne by the sponsor. In other words, the study is free.

172. Can I stop in the middle of the study?

Patients can stop participating in a study at any time and for any reason. Patients usually withdraw from studies only if they have a severe adverse reaction to the drug or if it fails to help them. (You should never begin a study if you are not convinced it is the right thing to do.)

173. What kind of results should I expect from a drug study?

Jim's story is fairly typical. He did not experience a dramatic improvement in his seizures, but they are now occurring less often and are less severe. He is somewhat better. Some patients do not benefit at all from a new drug, and a few get worse.

174. How do I know if there is a protocol drug that might help me?

If your seizures remain uncontrolled and your doctor has exhausted new treatment options, you should ask for a referral to a comprehensive epilepsy center. (See Appendix D.) There you will be evaluated to see if you fit the inclusion and exclusion criteria of the particular study. For example, in one of our studies, in order to be included a patient must be between 15 and 70 years old and have partial complex seizures at least three times a month. Patients are excluded if they are pregnant, have severe medical or psychiatric disease, abuse drugs or alcohol, or are noncompliant.

If you qualify for the study, the details will be explained to you, as well as potential risks, benefits, and costs. Then you can decide whether you want to participate.

175. What is informed consent?

Informed consent is an ethical concept that presumes an individual to be the best person to make a decision regarding his or her own care. Before you enroll in a study, the possible risks to your health, potential benefits from the drug, and alternatives to the study must be discussed with you. The FDA requires that you sign an informed consent form in order to begin a drug trial.

176. What is an open label trial?

In many clinical trials, the name and amount of experimental drug are known to the investigator and the patient. This is an open label trial.

(A study in which the investigator or patient does not know whether an investigational drug or placebo is being used is a blinded trial.)

177. What is a placebo?

In certain drug study protocols, some patients receive active drug while others receive an inactive substance, or placebo. The placebo is designed to look like the study drug.

In a "single blind study," the doctor is aware which one the patient is taking, but the patient is not. In a "double blind study," neither the doctor nor the patient knows. Records are kept in code. At the end of the trial, the "blind is broken" and the results are analyzed by the manufacturer. The seizure frequency of the two groups is compared to see whether the new drug helped patients more than the placebo.

178. What is a "placebo effect?"

For reasons that remain mysterious, under the proper circumstances some patients improve with anything new, usually temporarily. Sarah is a 20-year-old patient of mine with a behavior disorder and frequent seizures (as often as 26 times a month). After trials of seven different epilepsy drugs failed to control her seizures, she reluctantly entered a drug trial. The first phase of the study required her to begin with a placebo, or sugar pill. When she returned for follow-up a month later, Sarah exclaimed she had not had one seizure! According to her mother, even her behavior was much improved. She had responded to the power of suggestion, not to a miracle drug.

179. Will my doctor be upset if I don't participate?

You should not feel any pressure to enter a drug study. If you are an appropriate candidate, it is natural for your doctor to encourage you.

(I have been frustrated by one of my patients who continues to have many seizures a month. She refuses to try any new medication because of the "risks." She does not seem to understand that there are also real risks to her continued seizures. I think she would do much better with a protocol medication. Maybe someday she will change her mind and we will find out.)

180. Are there any other options for Jim since the new drug doesn't work?

Several investigational epilepsy drugs are currently being tested in the United States. (See Appendix B.) Jim is comfortable now with his improvement and not ready to try something new. However, if he would like to, he can choose to enroll in a different drug trial.

Another option for patients with intractable epilepsy is the vagal pacemaker, a new device to control seizures. Similar to a cardiac pacemaker, this device is implanted under the skin in the chest. A small wire connects to the vagus nerve, a large nerve in the neck. The wire sends an electric current to the nerve, which then stimulates the brain. This device has been approved by the FDA and is available at comprehensive epilepsy centers.

15. Who Else Can Help?

Sandy had seizures since infancy. She described a "feeling from behind," like a "wave." Then she would become confused. On rare occasions, she had a convulsion. Over the years, she tried nine medications to control her seizures, and she still had about three seizures a month. Her electroencephalographs (EEGs) and magnetic resonance imaging (MRI) pointed to a seizure focus in her right temporal lobe.

When I recommended epilepsy surgery, she became frightened and didn't return to see me for nearly a year. It was only because of the repeated urging of her friend who had already had seizure surgery that she came back. Last year, she consented to a right temporal lobectomy. Today, she is seizure-free.

181. Should I go to a support group?

Not everyone has a knowledgeable, supportive friend like Sandy. If your seizures are causing problems at home, at work, or with transportation, you may want to attend a support group to benefit from the experience of other people with epilepsy. Without her friend's encouragement, Sandy would have never returned for another look at surgery.

A support group can be very helpful. Others in your community with epilepsy are likely to know which pharmacy has the lowest medication prices, have opinions on the best epilepsy doctors, and recommend the most responsive social agencies.

Many people also feel better when they learn that others suffer the same problems. In some cases, patients discover that their epilepsy is much milder than others in the support group.

If your seizures are well-controlled and epilepsy does not interfere with your life, you do not need a support group. You may wish to go in order to help others become as well-adjusted as you are.

182. I would be more comfortable talking to people with epilepsy outside my community. What can I do?

The Epilepsy Foundation (EF) sponsors a national educational conference each year for people with epilepsy, families, and health professionals. Contact the EF for details.

183. What about a counselor?

Many patients benefit from discussing their problems with a clinical psychologist or other trained counselor. According to one epilepsy specialist, nearly all patients with epilepsy and their families require counseling sometime along the way. Modern life is stressful, and uncontrolled seizures compound daily problems. Not being able to drive or work puts pressure on people with epilepsy and their families. Sometimes a psychologist or other professional can help patients deal more effectively with these challenges. Counselors may also be available at school or church.

184. What about a social worker?

Comprehensive epilepsy centers and hospitals employ social workers who can assist you with transportation and funding. Some patients may qualify for disability or Medicaid, but need help in the application process. Special transportation may be available that you may not know about. A social worker is an excellent community resource.

185. My doctor is always so busy, and I have so many questions! Whom do I ask?

Not all of your questions need to be answered by your doctor. In my office, trained nurses and medical office assistants answer most patient questions over the telephone. We also distribute educational pamphlets that discuss common problems such as epilepsy first aid, neurologic testing, and driving. I try to answer difficult or complex questions during office visits.

For more general questions, find the address of your local EF affiliate in Appendix C and ask about an epilepsy education class. See if there is a comprehensive epilepsy center nearby. (See Appendix D.) Your pharmacist will be happy to provide printed information about your epilepsy medication.

Check the bibliography for books that interest you. Try the public library. Excellent pamphlets, books, and videos are available from the EF catalog. The

EF also maintains an outstanding library and can provide referrals over the phone.

Support groups and epilepsy societies exist all over the world. (See Appendix G.) There are even World Wide Web pages on the Internet devoted to epilepsy and the human brain. (Check Appendix H for Internet addresses.)

186. What about vocational rehabilitation (VR)?

If you are unemployed, ask your doctor for a referral to VR. They will assess your skills and may arrange job training. VR can determine whether it is practical for you to work and help you find an appropriate job.

187. I have trouble taking care of myself, doing chores, and looking after the children, particularly since I can't drive anywhere, but I can't afford any help. What can I do?

One of my patients with severe memory problems obtained considerable home assistance for her new baby from the members of her church. Many congregations feel that it is their responsibility to care for the needy. Talk to your pastor or rabbi about your situation. At the very least, you may find some spiritual support.

188. What about legal help? I'm concerned that I may lose my job because of epilepsy.

Some attorneys provide free (pro bono) assistance as a public service. Contact your EF affiliate for information on local legal resources.

189. I've been seeing my family doctor for five years. He has tried me on several drugs but I keep having seizures. Isn't there anything else I can do?

It may be time for a referral to a neurologist who specializes in epilepsy management or to a comprehensive epilepsy center. (See Appendix D.) There have been significant advances in the last ten years in the management of epilepsy and the newest treatments are only available at epilepsy centers. Tell your doctor how much you appreciate working with him and ask whether you might benefit from seeing an epilepsy specialist. If your seizures are not controlled, chances are your doctor is as frustrated as you and will embrace this suggestion.

16. NONEPILEPTIC SEIZURES

When I met Katherine at the hospital, she was 20 years old, four months pregnant, and homeless. She had a history of depression, sexual and physical abuse, and three suicide attempts. She was separated from her husband and lived in a shelter for pregnant women. Several months earlier, Kathy was injured in a fight with her boyfriend. Her father was going to testify against the boyfriend but died of a heart attack while waiting for the trial. Her mother blamed Kathy for her father's death, became depressed, and committed suicide. Then Kathy was hospitalized for depression. The workers at the shelter said she had behavior problems and was difficult to manage.

Kathy's seizures began at the age of 5, but she received no treatment until age 18. Eventually, one doctor prescribed carbamazepine (Tegretol®), which made her wobbly and sleepy. Then she began divalproex sodium (Depakote®), which she tolerated better, but she continued to have breakthrough seizures. When Kathy discovered she was pregnant, at ten weeks, she stopped taking the medication. Her seizure frequency increased, resulting in two emergency room visits and now this hospital admission to the epilepsy monitoring unit. Kathy's neurologic exam and magnetic resonance imaging (MRI) were normal.

Over several days, we recorded five of her seizures on the closed circuit television and electroencephalograph (CCTV/EEG) monitoring equipment. She lost consciousness during each spell. In one of them, she had dramatic jerking, pelvic thrusting, grimacing, and crying. Not one of the EEGs showed any epileptic activity. I explained to her that she had nonepileptic seizures, or pseudoseizures. Kathy had trouble accepting that her spells resulted from the significant social stresses in her life and not from epilepsy.

190. What is a pseudoseizure?

Some patients experience spells that resemble epileptic seizures. The patients may stare and be unresponsive, or even jerk and salivate. In epileptic seizures, there is always a distinctive discharge from neurons in the brain. In pseudo-seizures, the brain waves reveal no epileptic activity.

191. How can you tell if a patient is having a pseudo-seizure or an epileptic seizure?

Sometimes an experienced neurologist can tell by watching the patient closely. Certain types of behaviors are rare in true epileptic seizures, but far more common in nonepileptic ones. A more reliable method is to monitor the patient on CCTV/EEG and record the spells. Then the videotapes can be studied in detail as well as the EEG. Using this method, we are able to accurately diagnose 90 percent of patients.

192. Why would someone fake a seizure?

In most cases, the patient is unaware that the seizure is not epileptic. To the patient, the seizure is real. Most of these patients experience significant psychosocial stress in their lives and have limited coping skills and poor family support. Katherine is a typical example of the type of person who is at risk for developing nonepileptic seizures. (Because psychological problems are often the underlying problem, pseudoseizures are sometimes called psychogenic seizures.)

193. What would make you suspect a patient has pseudoseizures?

Sometimes the clinical history is suggestive, with an unusual time course, bizarre seizure types, or failure to respond to antiepileptic medications, especially when seen in a patient who has obvious psychological problems. It was peculiar, for example, that Kathy had seizures throughout most of her life, but no medications were prescribed until she was 18 years old. She was also in a high risk group, women of childbearing age with a history of physical and sexual abuse.

194. I have never heard of pseudoseizures. How common a problem is it?

In my specialized epilepsy practice over the last five years, I have seen 160 cases, so it is not rare. But the vast majority of patients with seizures have epilepsy, not pseudoseizures.

195. Can pseudoseizures occur in children?

Yes. They can occur at most any age. (I have a few patients with pseudoseizures in their eighties.)

196. Are there other causes of pseudoseizures besides psychiatric disease?

Yes. Sometimes patients have other medical problems that mimic epileptic seizures. They can be challenging to diagnose. For example, I took care of one patient with diabetes who would occasionally feel sleepy, slump over, and become stiff. When we monitored her on the epilepsy unit, her blood sugars were normal and there was no epileptic activity on the EEG. Initially, the problem appeared psychological. However, after studying her more closely, we discovered that she had a severe diabetic autonomic neuropathy. Unexpected drops in blood pressure lowered the flow of oxygen to her brain, causing her to pass out. In this case, treatment was medical, not psychological.

197. Do epilepsy medications help treat pseudoseizures?

No. Antiepileptic medications such as carbamazepine (Tegretol®), divalproex sodium (Depakote®), phenytoin (Dilantin®), or phenobarbital do not control pseudoseizures. That is one great value of making the correct diagnosis, because patients can be protected from the cost and health risks of taking medications they do not need. (Kathy suffered side effects from carbamazepine and her baby risked birth defects from valproic acid. Both medications were intended to treat epilepsy, a disorder she did not have!)

198. How do you treat pseudoseizures?

The first part of treatment is making an accurate diagnosis. This can only be done reliably with the use of EEG and typically takes place at an epilepsy center. Once the diagnosis is made, it must be carefully explained to the patient and family. Epilepsy medication is slowly withdrawn. The patients must enter into therapy with a psychiatrist or psychologist. If the patients have significant psychiatric illness, such as depression or anxiety, the psychiatrist may prescribe specific medication, such as an antidepressant.

In my practice, I run a monthly group therapy session for patients with pseudoseizures, in which we discuss the diagnosis, evaluate psychosocial stressors, and keep track of the seizures. Many patients find support in knowing there are others with the same unusual problem.

199. Can a patient have both epileptic and nonepileptic seizures?

Yes, although this does not occur often. As you may imagine, these patients are difficult to treat. They require antiepileptic medications and psychotherapy.

My Health Record
PERSONAL MEDICAL HISTORY

Have you ever had any of the following problems? (If you do not know, check with family members and try to complete this list before you see your neurologist.)

Problems at birth? Premature? Low birth weight? Needed an incubator? _____

Problems with development? How old were you when you learned to walk and talk? _____

How much school did you complete? _____
_____

Did you require special classes? _____

Encephalitis (infection in the brain)? _____

Meningitis (infection in the coverings of the brain)? _____

Head injury with loss of consciousness? _____

Febrile seizures (seizures with fever as an infant)? _____

Family member with epilepsy? _____

Allergies to medications or injections? _____

Medical illness requiring hospitalization? _____

Psychiatric illness (depression, hallucinations)? _____

Problem with drugs or alcohol? _____

Surgery? _____

Can you describe your seizure? Ask a friend or family member to help you:

Do you have a warning? _____

Do you have a convulsion? _____

Do you stare? _____

Do you lose control of your urine? _____

Do you bite your tongue? _____

Are you tired after a seizure? _____

Do you have a headache afterwards? _____

How often do they occur? _____

Are they more frequent around the time of your period? _____

Do seizures happen only at night? _____

Does anything seem to trigger your seizures? _____

Write down the medications you take for epilepsy and when you take them:

TIME OF DAY	MEDICATION #1 (MG)	MEDICATION #2 (MG)	MEDICATION #3 (MG)
MORNING:			
NOON:			
SUPPER:			
BEDTIME:			

Do these medications completely control your seizures? Yes/No _____

Do these medications give you any troublesome side effects? Yes/No _____

If you do have side effects, what are they?

_____

Do you take any other medications for other health problems? List them here:

_____

_____

_____

Write down any medications you have tried for epilepsy in the past that did not work:

_____

If you have had any of the following tests, write down the results if you know them:

MRI: _____

CAT Scan: _____

EEG: _____

IMPORTANT TELEPHONE NUMBERS

1. Medical doctor:

2. Neurologist:

3. Pharmacist:

4. Supervisor at work:

5. Closest family member:

6. Friend who drives:

7. Person to call in emergency:

It is important to keep a seizure calendar.
Place an 'X' on the calendar if you have a seizure, an 'O' if you have an aura. Put an 'M' if you missed any medication.

	M	T	W	T	F	S	S
J							
A							
N							
U							
A							
R							
Y							

M	T	W	T	F	S	S

FEBRUARY

	M	T	W	T	F	S	S
M A R C H							

M	T	W	T	F	S	S

APRIL

M	T	W	T	F	S	S

MAY

M	T	W	T	F	S	S

JUNE

M	T	W	T	F	S	S

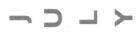

JULY

M	T	W	T	F	S	S

AUGUST

M	T	W	T	F	S	S

SEPTEMBER

M	T	W	T	F	S	S

OCTOBER

M	T	W	T	F	S	S

NOVEMBER

M	T	W	T	F	S	S

DECEMBER

Pharmaceutical and Medical Device Companies

MEDICATIONS, WEB SITES, AND CONTACT INFORMATION

Medications for the Treatment of Epilepsy

Brand Name (USA)	Generic
Carbatrol	carbamazepine extended release
Celontin	methsuximide
Cerebyx	fosphenytoin
Dilantin	phenytoin
Depakene	valproic acid
Depakote	divalproex sodium
Diamox	acetazolamide
Felbatol	felbamate
Gabitril	tiagabine
Keppra	levetiracetam
Klonopin	clonazepam
Lamictal	lamotrigine
Mebaral	mephobarbital
Mysoline	primidone
Neurontin	gabapentin
Phenobarbital	phenobarbital
Tegretol	carbamazepine
Tegretol XR	carbamazepine extended release
Topamax	topiramate
Tranzene	clorazepate
Trileptal	oxcarbazepine
Zarontin	ethosuximide
Zonegran	zonisamide

Investigational Antiepileptic Medications*

Brand Name (USA)	Generic
pending	ganaxolone
pending	harkoseride
pending	losigamone
pending	nefiracetam
pending	pregabalin
pending	remacemide
pending	retigabine
pending	valrocemide

*These are research drugs for the treatment of epilepsy in various phases of development. As of March 2002, they are not approved by the FDA.

Information Resources

(These numbers and web sites may help your doctor obtain information about pharmaceutical company–sponsored indigent programs or answer specific inquiries about medications.)

○ Abbott Laboratories (Depacon, Depakote), www.abbott.com, (800) 222-6883

○ Cephalon Professional Services (Gabitril), www.cephalon.com, (800) 896-5855

○ Cyberonics, Inc. (Vagal Nerve Stimulator), www.cyberonics.com, (800) 332-1375

○ Elan Pharmaceuticals (Zonegran), www.elan.com, (650) 877-0900

○ GlaxoSmithKline (Lamictal), www.gsk.com, (800) 722-9292

○ Novartis (Tegretol, Tegretol XR, Trileptal), www.novartis.com, (888) 644-8585

○ Ortho-McNeil Pharmaceuticals (Topamax), www.ortho-mcneil.com, (800) 682-6532

○ Pfizer (Celontin, Dilantin, Neurontin, Zarontin), www.pfizer.com, (800) 223-0432

○ Roche Laboratories (Klonopin), www.roche.com, (800) 526-6367

○ Sanofi-Synthelabo (Mebaral), www.sanofi-synthelabous.com, (800) 446-6267

○ Shire US, Inc. (Carbatrol), www.shire.com, (800) 536-7878

○ UCB Pharma (Keppra), www.ucb.be, (800) 477-7877

○ Wallace Laboratories (Felbatol), www.wallacepharmaceuticals.com, (609) 655-6000

○ Wyeth (Diamox), www.wyeth.com, (800) 934-5556

APPENDIX C

Resource Guide

EPILEPSY FOUNDATION
4351 Garden City Drive
Landover, MD 20785
Information Service
(800) EF-1000
Administrative office
(301) 459-3700

AMERICAN EPILEPSY SOCIETY
638 Prospect Avenue
Hartford, CT 06105-4298
Tel: (203) 586-7505
Fax: (203) 586-7550

EPILEPSY FOUNDATION
National Epilepsy Library Database
(largest single source of information on
the social and medical aspects of
epilepsy in the world)
Tel: (800) EF-4050
Fax: (301) 577-4941

State Epilepsy Associations

**EPILEPSY FOUNDATION OF NORTH
AND CENTRAL ALABAMA**
701 37th Street, South, Suite 2
Birmingham, AL 35222
(205) 324-4222

**EPILEPSY FOUNDATION
OF SOUTH ALABAMA**
951 Government Street, Suite 201
Mobile, AL 36604
(251) 432-0970

EPILEPSY FOUNDATION OF ARIZONA
P.O. Box 25084
Phoenix, AZ 85002-5084
(602) 406-3581

**EPILEPSY FOUNDATION OF
NORTHERN CALIFORNIA**
1624 Franklin Street, Suite 900
Oakland, CA 94612-2124
(510) 893-6272

**EPILEPSY FOUNDATION OF SAN
DIEGO COUNTY**
2055 El Cajon Boulevard
San Diego, CA 92104
(619) 296-0161

**EPILEPSY FOUNDATION OF
LOS ANGELES, ORANGE,
SAN BERNARDINO AND
VENTURA COUNTIES**
577 West Century Boulevard, Suite 820
Los Angeles, CA 90045
(310) 670-2870

**EPILEPSY FOUNDATION OF
COLORADO, INC.**
234 Columbine Street, Suite 333
Denver, CO 80206
(303) 377-9774

EPILEPSY FOUNDATION OF CONNECTICUT, INC.
386 Main Street
Middletown, CT 06457
(860) 346-1924

EPILEPSY FOUNDATION OF DELAWARE
New Castle Corporate Commons
61 Corporate Circle
New Castle, DE 19720
(302) 324-4455

THE EPILEPSY FOUNDATION OF NORTHEAST FLORIDA, INC.
5209 San Jose Boulevard, Suite 101
Jacksonville, FL 32207
(904) 731-3752

SUB-UNIT
The Epilepsy Foundation of Northeast
Florida, Inc.
Volusia-Flagler Extension
P.O. Box 2854
Ormond Beach, FL 32175
(904) 947-3547

EPILEPSY FOUNDATION OF SOUTH FLORIDA, INC.
7300 North Kendall Drive, Suite 700
Miami, FL 33156
(305) 670-4949, ext. 211

SUB-UNIT
Epilepsy Services of Broward, Inc.
512 NE 3rd Avenue
Ft. Lauderdale, FL 33301
(954) 779-1509

SUB-UNIT
Epilepsy Foundation of Eastern Florida
3233 Commerce Place, Suite C
West Palm Beach, FL 33407-2032
(561) 478-6515

EPILEPSY FOUNDATION OF GEORGIA
100 Edgewood Avenue, Northeast,
Suite 1200
Atlanta, GA 30303
(404) 527-7155

SUB-UNIT
Epilepsy Foundation of NW Georgia,
Inc.
305 South Thornton Avenue, Suite 102
Dalton, GA 30720
(706) 226-1248

EPILEPSY FOUNDATION OF HAWAII
245 North Kukui Street, Suite 207
Honolulu, HI 96817-3921
(808) 528-3058

EPILEPSY FOUNDATION OF IDAHO
310 West Idaho
Boise, ID 83702
(208) 344-4340

SUB-UNIT
Epilepsy Foundation of Idaho
Eastern Idaho Outreach Office
480 Park Avenue, Suite 3A
Idaho Falls, ID 83402
(208) 529-3580

SUB-UNIT
Epilepsy Foundation of Idaho
North Idaho Office
2101 Lakewood Drive, Suite 234
Coeur d'Alene, ID 83814
(208) 765-9443

EPILEPSY FOUNDATION OF NORTH/CENTRAL ILLINOIS
321 West State Street, Suite 208
Rockford, IL 61101-1119
(815) 964-2689

SUB-UNIT
Epilepsy Foundation of North/
Central Illinois
DeKalb Office
626 Bethany Road
DeKalb, IL 60115
(815) 756-8554

**EPILEPSY FOUNDATION OF GREATER
CHICAGO**
20 East Jackson Boulevard, 13th Floor
Chicago, IL 60604
(312) 939-8622

**EPILEPSY ASSOCIATION OF SOUTH-
WESTERN ILLINOIS**
1931 West Main Street
Belleville, IL 62226
(618) 236-2181

**EPILEPSY FOUNDATION KENTUCK-
IANA**
501 East Broadway, Suite 110
Louisville, KY 40202
(502) 584-8817

**EPILEPSY FOUNDATION SOUTHEAST
LOUISIANA**
3701 Canal Street, Suite H
New Orleans, LA 70119
(208) 529-3580

**EPILEPSY FOUNDATION OF THE
CHESAPEAKE REGION**
Hampton Plaza
300 East Joppa Road, Suite 1103
Towson, MD 21286
(410) 828-7700

SUB-UNIT
Epilepsy Association of Maryland
Southern Maryland Office
132 Holiday Court, Suite 211
Annapolis, MD 21401-7054
(410) 266-7941

SUB-UNIT
Epilepsy Association of Maryland
Western Maryland Office
174 Thomas Johnson Drive, Suite 202
Frederick, MD 21702-4334
(301) 695-9505

SUB-UNIT
Epilepsy Association of Maryland
Silver Spring Office
1738 Elton Road, Suite 320
Silver Spring, MD 20903
(301) 431-7740

SUB-UNIT
Epilepsy Association of Maryland
Eastern Shore Office
921 Mount Hermon Road
Salisbury, MD 21801
(410) 543-0665

SUB-UNIT
Epilepsy Foundation of the Chesapeake
Region
Virginia Office
4031 University Drive, Suite 110
Fairfax, VA 22020-3409
(703) 385-8501

SUB-UNIT
Epilepsy Association of Maryland
Washington, D.C. Office
4224 6th Street SE
Washington, DC 20032
(202) 561-6114

**EPILEPSY FOUNDATION OF MASSA-
CHUSETTS AND RHODE ISLAND**
95 Berkeley Street, Suite 409
Boston, MA 02116
(617) 542-2292

**EPILEPSY FOUNDATION
OF MICHIGAN**
26211 Central Park Boulevard,
Suite 100
Southfield, MI 48076
(248) 351-7979

EPILEPSY FOUNDATION OF MINNESOTA
2356 University Avenue W., Suite 405
St. Paul, MN 55114
(651) 646-8675

SUB-UNIT
Epilepsy Foundation of Minnesota
Southeast Minnesota Office
903 Center Street West
Rochester, MN 55902
(507) 287-2103

SUB-UNIT
Epilepsy Foundation of Minnesota
West Central Minnesota Office
14 7th Avenue, North
St. Cloud, MN 56301
(612) 259-4036

EPILEPSY FOUNDATION OF MISSISSIPPI
P.O. Box 16232
Jackson, MS 39236
(601) 362-2761

SUB-UNIT
Epilepsy Foundation of Northeast
Mississippi
102 North Main Street, Suite B
Ripley, MS 38663
(662) 837-8626

EPILEPSY FOUNDATION OF KANSAS AND WESTERN MISSOURI
6550 Troost, Suite B
Kansas City, MO 64131-1272
(816) 444-2800

EPILEPSY FOUNDATION OF THE ST. LOUIS REGION
7100 Oakland Avenue
St. Louis, MO 63117-1881
(314) 645-6969

SUB-UNIT
Epilepsy Foundation of Southern
Illinois
1100 D. South 42nd Street
Mt. Vernon, IL 62864
(618) 244-6680

EPILEPSY FOUNDATION OF NEW JERSEY
429 River View Plaza
Trenton, NJ 08611
(609) 392-4900

SUB-UNIT
Epilepsy Foundation of New Jersey
North Jersey Office
513 West Mt. Pleasant Avenue, Suite 200
Livingston, NJ 07039
(973) 992-5900

SUB-UNIT
Epilepsy Foundation of New Jersey
Shore Area Office
Lions Head Office Park
35 Beaverson Boulevard, Suite 8A
Brick, NJ 08723
(732) 262-8020

SUB-UNIT
Epilepsy Foundation of New Jersey
South Jersey Office
216 Hadden Avenue
Westmont, NJ -8108
(856) 858-5900

EPILEPSY ASSOCIATION OF ROCHESTER, SYRACUSE, AND BINGHAMTON
1000 Elmwood Avenue
Rochester, NY 14620
(716) 442-4430

SUB-UNIT
Epilepsy Assocation of Rochester,
Syracuse, and Binghamton
Field Office—Broom County
24 Prospect Avenue, Box 12
Binghamton, NY 13901
(607) 722-6822

EPILEPSY FOUNDATION OF LONG ISLAND, INC.
550 Stewart Avenue
Garden City, NY 11530
(516) 739-7733

SUB-UNIT
Epilepsy Foundation of Long Island, Inc.
2100 Middle Country Road
First Floor, Room 106A
Centereach, NY 11720
(516) 467-3989

EPILEPSY FOUNDATION OF NEW YORK CITY
305 7th Avenue, 12th Floor
New York, NY 10001
(212) 633-2930

EPILEPSY FOUNDATION OF SOUTHERN NEW YORK
One Blue Hill Plaza, Box 1745
Pearl River, NY 10965
(845) 627-0627

SUB-UNIT
Epilepsy Foundation of Southern New York
Field Office—Orange County
726 East Main Street
Middletown, NY 10940
(845) 344-0450

EPILEPSY FOUNDATION OF NORTHEASTERN NEW YORK
Three Washington Square
Albany, NY 12205
(518) 456-7501

EPILEPSY FOUNDATION OF NORTH CAROLINA, INC.
3001 Spring Forest Road
Raleigh, NC 27616-2817
(919) 876-7788

SUB-UNIT
Epilepsy Foundation of North Carolina, Inc.
Western Field Office
200 Hawthorne Lane
Charlotte, NC 28204
(704) 377-EANC

EPILEPSY FOUNDATION OF CENTRAL OHIO
454 East Main Street, Suite 250
Columbus, OH 43215-5380
(614) 228-4401

EPILEPSY COUNCIL OF GREATER CINCINNATI
3 Centennial Plaza
895 Central Avenue, Suite 550
Cincinnati, OH 45202
(513) 721-2905

SUB-UNIT
Epilepsy Council of Greater Cincinnati
Warren County, OH
570 North State, Route 741
Lebanon, OH 45036
(513) 925-2250

SUB-UNIT
Epilepsy Council of Greater Cincinnati
Eastern and Central Kentucky
205 Main Street
Williamstown, KY 41097
(606) 824-6699

EPILEPSY FOUNDATION OF WESTERN OHIO
7523 Brandt Pike
Dayton, OH 45424
(937) 233-2500

EPILEPSY FOUNDATION OF NORTHEAST OHIO
2800 Euclid Avenue, Room 450
Cleveland, OH 44115
(216) 579-1330

SUB-UNIT
Epilepsy Foundation of Northeast Ohio
Lorain County Office
1875 North Ridge Road, Suite E
Lorain, OH 44005
(216) 277-6692

EPILEPSY CENTER OF NORTHWEST OHIO
1251 South Reynolds Road, PMB 323
Toledo, OH 43615
(800) 377-6226

EPILEPSY FOUNDATION OF OREGON
619 S.W. 11th Avenue, Suite 225
Portland, OR 97205
(503) 228-7651

EPILEPSY FOUNDATION OF EASTERN PENNSYLVANIA
Seven Benjamin Franklin Parkway
6th Floor Front
Philadelphia, PA 19103-1208
(215) 523-9180

SUB-UNIT
Epilepsy Foundation of Eastern
Pennsylvania
Northeast Subunit
P.O. Box 26
Tunkhannock, PA 18657
(570) 996-0776

EPILEPSY FOUNDATION OF WESTERN AND CENTRAL PENNSYLVANIA
Vocational Rehab Center
1323 Forbes Avenue, Suite 102
Pittsburgh, PA 15219
(412) 261-5880

EPILEPSY FOUNDATION CENTRAL PENNSYLVANIA
900 South Arlington Avenue, Suite 236
Harrisburg, PA 17109
(717) 541-0301

SOCIEDAD PUERTORRIQUENA DE EPILEPSIA
Hospital Ruiz Soler
Calle Marginal Final
Bayamon, Puerto Rico 00959
(787) 782-6200

EPILEPSY FOUNDATION OF SOUTH CAROLINA
652 Bush River Road, Suite 211
Columbia, SC 29210
(803) 798-8502

EPILEPSY FOUNDATION OF WEST TENNESSEE
70 TimberCreek #1
Cordova, TN 38018
(901) 624-7148

SUB-UNIT
Epilepsy Foundation of West Tennessee
Field Office
1979 St. John
Dyersburg, TN 38024
(901) 286-0044

EPILEPSY FOUNDATION OF SOUTHEAST TENNESSEE
744 McCallie Avenue, Suite 301
Chattanooga, TN 37403
(423) 756-1771

EPILEPSY FOUNDATION OF EAST TENNESSEE
P.O. Box 3156
Knoxville, TN 37927
(865) 522-4991

EPILEPSY FOUNDATION OF MIDDLE TENNESSEE
2002 Richard Jones Road, #C202
Nashville, TN 37215
(615) 269-7091

SUB-UNIT
Epilepsy Foundation of Middle Tennessee
South Central Regional Office
319 Bethany Lane
Shelbyville, TN 37160
(615) 684-5222

SUB-UNIT
Epilepsy Foundation of Middle Tennessee
Clarksville Regional Office
1241 Highway Drive
Clarksville, TN 37040
(615) 648-9675

SUB-UNIT
Epilepsy Foundation of Middle Tennessee
Upper Cumberland Regional Office
122 South Madison Avenue
Cookeville, TN 38501
(615) 372-8082

SUB-UNIT
Epilepsy Foundation of Middle Tennessee
Gallatin Regional Office
450 West Main Street, Building A, Suite 1
Gallatin, TN 37066
(615) 452-1869 or (615) 500-8277

DALLAS EPILEPSY ASSOCIATION
2906 Swiss Avenue
Dallas, TX 75204
(214) 823-8809

EPILEPSY FOUNDATION OF GREATER NORTH TEXAS
2906 Swiss Avenue
Dallas, TX 75204
(214) 823-8809

SUB-UNIT
Epilepsy Foundation of Greater North Texas
Mesquite Office
1035 Military Parkway
Mesquite, TX 75149
(972) 290-9922

SUB-UNIT
Epilepsy Foundation of Greater North Texas
700 Olympic Plaza
Tyler, TX 75701-1955
(903) 535-6897

EPILEPSY FOUNDATION OF SOUTHEAST TEXAS
2650 Fountain View, Suite 316
Houston, TX 77057
(713) 789-6295

SUB-UNIT
Epilepsy Foundation of Southeast Texas
855 East Florida Avenue, Suite 117A
Beaumont, TX 77705
(409) 839-2950

EPILEPSY FOUNDATION OF CENTRAL AND SOUTH TEXAS
10615 Perrin Beitel, Suite 602
San Antonio, TX 78217
(210) 653-5353

EPILEPSY FOUNDATION OF VERMONT
P.O. Box 6292
Rutland, VT 05702
(802) 775-1686

EPILEPSY ASSOCIATION OF VERMONT
Sulivan Hall
92 Ethan Allen Avenue
Colchester, VT 05446
(802) 655-4566

EPILEPSY FOUNDATION OF VIRGINIA
UVA Health Services Center
P.O. Box 800569
Charlottesville, VA 22908
(804) 924-8678

**EPILEPSY FOUNDATION OF WASHING-
TON**
3800 Aurora Avenue North, Suite 370
Seattle, WA 98103
(206) 547-4551

**EPILEPSY FOUNDATION OF SOUTH-
EAST WISCONSIN**
735 N. Water Street, Suite 701
Milwaukee, WI 53202
(414) 271-0110

**EPILEPSY FOUNDATION OF WESTERN
WISCONSIN**
1812 Brackett Avenue, Suite 5
Eau Claire, WI 54701
(715) 834-4455

**EPILEPSY FOUNDATION OF SOUTH
CENTERAL WISCONSIN**
7617 Mineral Point Road
Madison, WI 53717-1623
(608) 833-8888

**EPILEPSY FOUNDATION OF CENTRAL
AND NORTHEAST WISCONSIN**
1004 First Street, Suite 5
Stevens Point, WI 54481-2627
(414) 730-1160

SUB-UNIT
Epilepsy Foundation of Central and
Northeast Wisconsin
Wausau Office
903 North 2nd Street
Wausau, WI 54403
(715) 845-2328

SUB-UNIT
Epilepsy Foundation of Central and
Northeast Wisconsin
Appleton Office
1800 Appleton Road
Menasha, WI 54952
(920) 968-3000

**EPILEPSY FOUNDATION OF SOUTHERN
WISCONSIN, INC.**
205 North Main Street, Suite 106
Janesville, WI 53545
(608) 755-1821

SUB-UNIT
Epilepsy Foundation of Southern
Wisconsin, Inc.
Grant, Iowa, and Crawford Counties
P.O. Box 213
Lancaster, WI 53813
(608) 723-4488

SUB-UNIT
Epilepsy Foundation of Southern
Wisconsin, Inc.
Racine and Kenosha Counties
P.O. Box 1016
Kenosha, WI 53141-1016
(262) 605-3352

Other Resources

**ASSOCIATION FOR THE CARE OF
CHILDREN'S HEALTH**
3615 Wisconsin Avenue
Washington, DC 20016
(202) 244-1801

**ASSOCIATION FOR CHILDREN
AND ADULTS WITH LEARNING
DISABILITIES**
4156 Library Road
Pittsburgh, PA 15234
(412) 341-1515

**ASSOCIATION FOR RETARDED CITI-
ZENS**
2501 Avenue J
Arlington, TX 76011
(871) 640-0204

CHILDREN'S DEFENSE FUND
25 E Street, N.W.
Washington, DC 20001
(202) 628-8787

**COUNCIL FOR EXCEPTIONAL CHIL-
DREN**
1920 Association Drive
Reston, VA 22091-1589
(703) 620-3660

**EPILEPSY CONCERN INTERNATIONAL
SERVICE GROUP**
Executive Director
1282 Wynnewood Drive
West Palm Beach, FL 33417
(407) 683-0044

EPILEPSY INFORMATION SERVICE
Medical Center Boulevard
Winston-Salem, NC 27157-1078
(800) 642-0500

**EQUAL EMPLOYMENT OPPORTUNITY
COMMISSION (EEOC)**
1801 L Street, N.W.
Washington, DC 20507
(800) 669-EEOC

JOSEPH P. KENNEDY FOUNDATION
1350 New York Avenue, N.W., Suite
500
Washington, DC 20005
(202) 393-1250

KIDS ON THE BLOCK
9385 C. Gerwig Lane
Columbia, MD 21046
(301) 368-KIDS

MEDIC ALERT FOUNDATION U.S.
2323 Colorado
Turlock, CA 95382
(800) 432-5378

**NATIONAL ASSOCIATION OF EPILEPSY
CENTERS**
5775 Wayzata Boulevard
Minneapolis, MN 55416
(952) 525-4526

**NATIONAL FOUNDATION FOR BRAIN
RESEARCH**
Suite 300
1250 24th Street N.W.
Washington, DC 20037
(202) 293-5453

**NATIONAL HEAD INJURY FOUNDA-
TION**
1776 Massachusetts Avenue N.W., #100
Washington, DC 20036-1904
(800) 444-6443

**NATIONAL INFORMATION CENTER
FOR CHILDREN AND YOUTH WITH
DISABILITIES**
Box 1492
Washington, DC 20013-1492
(800) 695-0285

**NATIONAL INSTITUTE OF NEUROLOG-
ICAL DISORDERS AND STROKE**
Office of Scientific and Health Reports
Box 5801
Bethesda, MD 20892
(800) 352-9424

**NATIONAL TUBEROUS SCLEROSIS
ASSOCIATION, INC.**
8181 Professional Place, Suite 110
Landover, Maryland 20785-2226
(800) 225-NTSA

OFFICE ON THE AMERICANS WITH DISABILITIES ACT
Civil Rights Division
U.S. Department of Justice
Box 66118
Washington, DC 20035-6118
(202) 514-0301

RESOURCES FOR CHILDREN WITH SPECIAL SKILLS
200 Park Avenue South, Suite 816
New York, NY 10003
(212) 677-4650

SIBLING INFORMATION CENTER
Department of Educational Psychology
Box U-64
The University of Connecticut
Storrs, CT 06268
(203) 486-4031

SIBLINGS FOR SIGNIFICANT CHANGE
823 United Nations Plaza, Room 808
New York, NY 10017
(212) 420-0776

THE WILL ROGERS INSTITUTE
785 Mamaroneck Avenue
White Plains, NY 10605
(914) 761-5550

THE CHARLIE FOUNDATION TO HELP CURE PEDIATRIC EPILEPSY
501 10th Street
Santa Monica, California 90402
(800) FOR-KETO ((800)367-5386)

THE EPILEPSY EDUCATION AND CONTROL ACTIVITIES DATABASE
(for health care professionals)
Centers for Disease Control and Prevention
National Center for Chronic Disease Prevention and Health Promotion
Technical Information Services Branch
4770 Buford Hwy, NE, MS-K13
Atlanta, Georgia 30341-3724
(404) 488-5080

National Association of Comprehensive Epilepsy Centers

EPILEPSY CENTER
Barrow Neurological Institute
St. Joseph's Hospital and Medical Center
350 West Thomas Road
Phoenix, AZ 85013-4496
David Blum, M.D.
(602) 406-3886

ARIZONA COMPREHENSIVE EPILEPSY PROGRAM
University Medical Center
1501 North Campbell
Tucson, AZ 85724
David M. Labiner, M.D.
(520) 694-4564

REED NEURO RESEARCH CENTER
Department of Neurology
UCLA School of Medicine
710 Westwood Plaza, Room 1250
Los Angeles, CA 90095
Marc Nuwer, M.D.
(310) 825-5745

EPILEPSY CENTER
University of California–San Diego
200 West Arbor Drive
San Diego, CA 92103
Vincent Iragui, M.D., Ph.D.
(619) 543-5302

EPILEPSY CENTER
University of California–San Francisco
400 Parnassus Avenue
Box 0138, Room 889
San Francisco, CA 94143
Kenneth Laxer, M.D.
(415) 476-6337

SACRAMENTO COMPREHENSIVE EPILEPSY PROGRAM
10 Congress Street, Suite 505
Pasadena, CA 91105
William W. Sutherling, M.D.
(626) 792-7300

STANFORD COMPREHENSIVE EPILEPSY CENTER
Department of Neurology
Stanford University Medical Center
300 Pasteur Drive, H3160
Stanford, CA 94305
Robert S. Fisher
(650) 725-6648

SECTION OF NEUROLOGY
Department of Medicine
Norwalk Hospital
Maple Street
Norwalk, CT 06851
Steven A. Jerrett, M.D.
(203) 852-2400

COMPREHENSIVE EPILEPSY CENTER
Miami Children's Hospital
3100 South West 62nd Avenue
Miami, FL 33155
Michael S. Duchowny, M.D.
(305) 662-8342

DEPARTMENT OF NEUROLOGY
MCG Health, Inc.
Medical College of Augusta Georgia
1459 Laney Walker Boulevard
Augusta, GA 30912
Donald W. King, M.D.
(706) 721-3325

RUSH PRESBYTERIAN EPILEPSY
CENTER
Department of Neurological Sciences
St. Luke's Medical Center
1653 West Congress Parkway
Chicago, IL 60612
Michael C. Smith, M.D.
(312) 942-5939

COMPREHENSIVE EPILEPSY PROGRAM
Indiana University Hospitals
550 North University Boulevard,
Room 1711
Indianapolis, IN 46202
Omkar N. Martkland, M.D.
(317) 274-0181

EPILEPSY CENTER
Via Christi Regional Medical Center
St. Francis Campus
929 North St. Francis
Wichita, KS 67214
Kore Liow, M.D.
(316) 268-8500

COMPREHENSIVE EPILEPSY
CENTER
Beth Israel Hospital
330 Brookline Avenue
Boston, MA 02215
Dr. Donald Schomer, M.D.
(617) 667-3999

✳ MARYLAND EPILEPSY CENTER
Department of Neurology
University of Maryland Hospital
22 South Greene Street
Baltimore, MD 21201-1595
Dr. Allan Krumholz, M.D.
(410) 328-0697

COMPREHENSIVE EPILEPSY
PROGRAM
Henry Ford Hospital
2799 West Grand Boulevard
Detroit, MI 48202
Gregory L. Barkley, M.D.
(313) 916-3922

MINNESOTA EPILEPSY GROUP
United Hospital
310 North Smith Avenue, Suite 300
St. Paul, MN 55102
John R. Gates, M.D.
(651) 220-5290

MINCEP EPILEPSY CARE
5775 Wayzata Boulevard, Suite 200
Minneapolis, MN 55416
Robert J. Gumnit, M.D.
(952) 525-2400

EPILEPSY CENTER
Mayo Clinic Foundation
200 First Street SW
Rochester, MN 55905
Gregory Cascino, M.D.
(507) 538-1032

COMPREHENSIVE EPILEPSY
CARE CENTER FOR CHILDREN
AND ADULTS, P.C.
St. Luke's North Medical Building
222 South Woods Mill Road, Suite 610
Chesterfield, MO 63017
William E. Rosenfeld, M.D.
(314) 453-9300

EPILEPSY CENTERS AT WASHINGTON
UNIVERSITY
Pediatric Epilepsy Center
St. Louis Children's Hospital
One Children's Place, Suite 12E47
St. Louis, MO 63110-1093
Edwin Trevathan, M.D., M.P.H.
(314) 454-4089

EPILEPSY CENTERS AT
WASHINGTON UNIVERSITY
Department of Neurology
660 South Euclid
St. Louis, MO 63110
Frank Gilliam, M.D.
(314) 362-7854

DEPARTMENT OF NEUROLOGY
University of North Carolina at
Chapel Hill
738 Burnett Womack Building, CB
7025
Chapel Hill, NC 27514
Robert Greenwood, MD
(919) 966-8160

COMPREHENSIVE EPILEPSY CENTER
Wake Forest University
Baptist Medical Center
Winston-Salem, NC 27157
William L. Bell, M.D.
(336) 716-0488

ALEGENT HEALTH
Immanuel Medical Center
6901 North 72nd Street
Omaha, NE 68122
Richard V. Andrews, M.D.
(402) 572-2566

**COLUMBIA COMPREHENSIVE
EPILEPSY CENTER**
The Neurological Institute
Columbia University
710 West 168th Street
New York, NY 10032
Marth Morrell, M.D.
(212) 305-1742

STRONG EPILEPSY CENTER
University of Rochester Medical Center
601 Elmwood Avenue, Box 673
Rochester, NY 14620-8673
Michel J. Berg, M.D.
(716) 275-8237

DEPARTMENT OF NEUROLOGY
Long Island Jewish Medical Center
270–05 76th Avenue
Research Building, Level C
New Hyde Park, NY 11040
Alan Ettinger, M.D.
(718) 470-7370

**NYU COMPREHENSIVE EPILEPSY
CENTER**
New York University
560 First Avenue
Rivergate, 4th Floor
New York, NY 10016
Orrin Devinsky, M.D.
(212) 598-6412

EPILEPSY PROGRAM
Montefiore Medical Center
Albert Einstein College of Medicine
111 East 210th Street
Bronx, NY 10467
Shlomo Shinnar M.D.
Solomon Moshe, M.D.
(718) 920-2906

**SUNY UPSTATE MEDICAL
UNIVERSITY**
700 East Adams Street
Syracuse, NY 13210
Robert L. Beach, M.D., Ph.D.
(315) 464-5360

**DEPARTMENT OF NEUROLOGY (PEDI-
ATRICS)**
Cleveland Clinic Foundation
9500 Euclid Avenue
Cleveland, OH 44106
Elaine Wyllie, M.D.
(216) 444-2200

**COMPREHENSIVE EPILEPSY
PROGRAM AT OHIO STATE
UNIVERSITY**
Children's Hospital
Ohio State University
700 Children's Drive
Columbus, OH 43205
Layne Moore, M.D.
(614) 722-4600

**COMPREHENSIVE EPILEPSY PRO-
GRAM OF UNIVERSITY CARE SYSTEM**
Department of Neurology
University Hospitals of Cleveland
11100 Euclid Avenue
Cleveland, OH 444106
Barbara Swartz, M.D., Ph.D.
(216) 844-3714

MOUNT CARMEL EPILEPSY CENTER
793 West State Street
Columbus, OH 43222
Jean Cibula, M.D.
(614) 234-5000

**COMPREHENSIVE EPILEPSY PRO-
GRAM AT OHIO STATE UNIVERSITY**
Children's Hospital
Ohio State University
700 Children's Drive
Columbus, OH 43205
Jullian Paolicchi, M.D.
(614) 722-4600

**COMPREHENSIVE OKLAHOMA PRO-
GRAM FOR EPILEPSY**
Department of Neurology
University of Oklahoma
Box 26901, Room 3SP203
920 Stanton L. Young Boulevard
Oklahoma City, OK 73190
Kalarickal Oommen, M.D.
(405) 271-4113 ext. 4602

COMPREHENSIVE EPILEPSY CENTER
Allegheny General Hospital
320 East North Avenue
Pittsburgh, PA 15212
James P. Valeriano, M.D.
(412) 321-2162

**JEFFERSON COMPREHENSIVE
EPILEPSY CENTER**
111 South 11th Street, Suite 4150
Philadelphia, PA 19107
Michael Sperling, M.D.
(215) 955-1222

**COMPREHENSIVE EPILEPSY
PROGRAM**
Rhode Island Hospital
110 Lockwood Street, Suite 342
Providence, RI 02903
Andrew Blum, M.D.
(401) 444-4345

**VANDERBILT UNIVERSITY EPILEPSY
PROGRAM**
Vanderbilt University
2100 Pierce Avenue, Suite 336
Nashville, TN 37212
Bassel Abou-Khalil, M.D.
(615) 936-2591

**LEBONHEUR CHILDREN'S MEDICAL
CENTER**
One Children's Plaza
Memphis, TN 38103
Frederick Boop, M.D.
(901) 572-3000

**UT SOUTHWESTERN EPILEPSY
CENTER**
Parkland Memorial Hospital
5201 Harry Hines Boulevard, 8th Floor
Dallas, TX 75235
Paul Van Ness, M.D.
(214) 590-8365

NEUROLOGICAL CLINIC OF TEXAS
Medical City Dallas Hospital
7777 Forest Lane, Suite B410
Dallas, TX 75320
Richard North, M.D.
(972) 566-7684

EPILEPSY CENTER
Baylor College of Medicine
One Baylor Plaza
Houston, TX 77030
Eli M. Mizrahi, M.D.
(713) 790-3105

TEXAS COMPREHENSIVE EPILEPSY PROGRAM
Department of Neurology
University of Texas at Houston
P.O. Box 20708
Houston, TX 77225-0708
James W. Wheless, M.D.
(713) 792-5777

NORTH TEXAS EPILEPSY CENTER
Department of Neurology
Baylor Medical Center Irving
2001 North MacArthur Boulevard,
Suite 500A
Irving, TX 75061
Henry G. Raroque, Jr., M.D.
(972) 251-1519

THE EPILEPSY CENTER/SEIZURE CLINIC
Presbyterian Hospital of Dallas
8200 Walnut Hill
Dallas, TX 75231
Jay Harvey, M.D.
(214) 345-7980

EPILEPSY INSTITUTE OF VIRGINIA
Department of Neurology
Virginia Commonwealth
Box 980599
Richmond, VA 23298-0599
Jack Pellock, M.D.
(804) 828-9869

COMPREHENSIVE EPILEPSY PROGRAM
Department of Neurology
University of Virginia Health Sciences
Center
P.O. Box 800394
Charlottesville, VA 22908
Nathan B. Fountain, M.D.
(804) 243-6281

SWEDISH MEDICAL CENTER
801 Broadway, Suite 830
Seattle, WA 98122
Allen Wyler, M.D.
(206) 386-3882

MARSHFIELD EPILEPSY PROGRAM
Department of Neurosciences
Marshfield Clinic
1000 North Oaks Avenue
Marshfield, WI 54449-5777
Kevin H. Ruggles, M.D.
(715) 387-5998

Driving and Epilepsy

STATE	SEIZURE-FREE PERIOD	PHYSICIANS MUST REPORT?
Alabama	6 months	no
Alaska	6 months	no
Arizona	3 months	no
Arkansas	1 year	no
California	varies	yes
Colorado	not set	no
Connecticut	not set	no
Delaware	not set	yes
District of Columbia	1 year	no
Florida	6 months	no
Georgia	6 months	no
Hawaii	1 year	no
Idaho	1 year	no
Illinois	not set	no
Indiana	not set	no
Iowa	6 months	no
Kansas	6 months	no
Kentucky	3 months	no
Louisiana	6 months	no
Maine	3 months	no
Maryland	3 months	no
Massachusetts	6 months	no
Michigan	6 months	no
Minnesota	6 months	no
Mississippi	1 year	no
Missouri	6 months	no
Montana	not set	no
Nebraska	3 months	no
Nevada	3 months	yes
New Hampshire	1 year	no
New Jersey	1 year	yes
New Mexico	1 year	no
New York	1 year	no
North Carolina	6–12 months	no

STATE	SEIZURE-FREE PERIOD	PHYSICIANS MUST REPORT?
North Dakota	6 months	no
Ohio	not set	no
Oklahoma	6 months	no
Oregon	6 months	yes
Pennsylvania	6 months	yes
Puerto Rico	not set	no
Rhode Island	18 months	no
South Carolina	6 months	no
South Dakota	6–12 months	no
Tennessee	6 months	no
Texas	6 months	no
Utah	3 months	no
Vermont	not set	no
Virginia	6 months	no
Washington	6 months	no
West Virginia	1 year	no
Wisconsin	3 months	no
Wyoming	3–12 months	no

Epilepsy Summer Camps

For information about scholarships, contact the Epilepsy Foundation. (800) 332-1000

ALABAMA

CAMP CANDLELIGHT AT CAMP ASCCA, AGES 8–18
Epilepsy Foundation of South Alabama
Epilepsy Foundation of North and Central Alabama
(334) 432-0970
(205) 324-4222

ARIZONA

CAMP CANDLELIGHT, AGES 8–15
Epilepsy Society of Arizona
(602) 406-3581
(888) 768-2690

CALIFORNIA

CAMP QUEST, AGES 8–13
Epilepsy Foundation of San Diego County
(619) 296-0161

COLORADO

ROCKY MOUNTAIN EPILEPSY CAMP, AGES 9–18
Epilepsy Foundation of Colorado
(303) 377-9774

CONNECTICUT

EASTER SEALS CAMP HEMLOCKS, AGES 6–18
Epilepsy Foundation of Connecticut
(800) 899-3745

FLORIDA

BOGGY CREEK GANG, AGES 7–16
Epilepsy Foundation of Eastern Florida
Epilepsy Foundation of South Florida
(561) 478-6515
(305) 663-6819

GEORGIA

EPILEPSY FOUNDATION OF GEORGIA
(404) 527-7155

ILLINOIS

CAMP BLACKHAWK, AGES 8–16
Epilepsy Foundation of North and Central Illinois
Epilepsy Foundation of Greater Chicago
(815) 964-2689
(618) 236-2181

CAMP ROEHR, AGES 6–18
Epilepsy Foundation of Southwestern Illinois
(618) 236-2181

LOUISIANA

CAMP TECHFUNCTE, AGES 6–18
Epilepsy Foundation of Southeast Louisiana
(504) 486-6326

MARYLAND

CHESAPEAKE CENTER, AGES 8–13
Epilepsy Foundation of the Chesapeake
Region
(410) 828-7700
(800) 492-2523

MICHIGAN

CAMP STORER, AGES 8–16
Epilepsy Foundation of Michigan
(248) 351-2102
(800) 377-6226

CAMP POWLER, AGES 8–19
EPILEPSY FOUNDATION OF MICHIGAN
(248) 351-2102
(800) 377-6226

MINNESOTA

CAMP OZ, AGES 8–17
Epilepsy Foundation of Minnesota
(651) 646-1771

MISSISSIPPI

ALVIN P. FLANNES CAMP, AGES 9–14
Epilepsy Foundation of Mississippi
(601) 362-2761

MISSOURI

CAMP SHING (SHINING STAR),
AGES 6–17
Epilepsy Foundation of Kansas and
Western Missouri
(816) 444-2800
(800) 972-5163

NEW JERSEY

CAMP NOVA, AGES 8–25
Epilepsy Foundation of New Jersey
(609) 392-4900

NEW YORK

CYO SUMMER DAY CAMP, AGES 4–13
Epilepsy Foundation of New York City
(212) 633-2930
Camp EAGR, ages 8–15
Epilepsy Foundation of Rochester and
Syracuse Regions
(716) 442-4430
(800) 724-7930

OHIO

CAMP DREAM CATCHER, AGES 8–17
Epilepsy Foundation of Greater
Cincinnati
(513) 721-2905
(877) 804-2241

CAMP CARPE DIEM, AGES 7–14
Epilepsy Foundation of Central Ohio
(614) 228-4401
Adventure Camp at Camp Cheerful,
ages 7–16
Epilepsy Foundation of Northeast Ohio
(216) 579-1330

OREGON

CAMP WECAN, AGES 8–13
Epilepsy Foundation of Oregon
(503) 228-7651

PENNSYLVANIA

TEEN RETREAT/PRE-TEEN RETREAT,
AGES 13–19/8–12
Epilepsy Foundation of Southeastern
Pennsylvania
(215) 523-9180
(800) 887-7165

CAMP FROG, AGES 8–18
Epilepsy Foundation of Western
Pennsylvania
(412) 261-5880
(800) 361-5885

SOUTH CAROLINA

CAMP RIVER RUN, AGES 7–14
Epilepsy Foundation of South Carolina
(803) 926-0071

TENNESSEE

CAMP LAKEWOOD, AGES 7–16
Epilepsy Foundation of Southest
Tennessee
(423) 756-1771

TEXAS

CAMP SPIKE 'N' WAVE, AGES 8–14
Epilepsy Foundation of Southeast Texas
(713) 789-6295
Camp Kaleidoscope, ages 15–19
Epilepsy Foundation of Southeeast
Texas
(713) 789-6295

WASHINGTON

CAMP DISCOVERY, AGES 7–17
Epilepsy Foundation
(206) 547-4551

WISCONSIN

**CAMP PHOENIX AT PHANTOM LAKE
YMCA CAMP, AGES 8–15**
Epilepsy Foundation of South Central
Wisconsin
(608) 833-8888
(800) 657-4929

International Epilepsy Resources[1]

Member List for the International Bureau for Epilepsy

ARGENTINA

Chapter
Asociacion de Lucha contra la Epilepsia
Tucuman 3261
1189 Buenos Aires

AUSTRALIA

Chapter
National Epilepsy Association of
Australia
Suite 2B, 44–46 Oxford Street
P.O. Box 879
Epping, NSW 21210

AUSTRIA

Chapter
Epilepsie Dachverband Österreich
Wichtelgasse 55/17–19
1170 Wien

BELGIUM

Chapter
Les Amis de la Ligue Nationale Belge
contre l'Epilepsie
Avenue Albert 135
Brussels 1060

BRAZIL

Chapter
Brazilian Association for Epilepsy
Rua Botucatu 862
04023–900
Sao Paulo, SP

BULGARIA

Chapter
Association for Assistance of Patients
with Epilepsy
Mladost 1, Building 65
Ent. A, App 10
1784 Sofia

CANADA

Chapter
Epilepsy Canada
1470 Pccl Strcct, Suite 745
Montreal, Quebec H3A 1T1

CHILE

Chapter
Liga Chilena contra la Epilepsia
Partiotas Uruguayos 2236
Codigo Postal: 6501205
Santiago

---

1 An International Directory of Epilepsy Self-help Groups can be obtained by writing to: The
Self-help Commission of The International Bureau for Epilepsy, Box 21, 2100 AA Heemstede,
The Netherlands.

COLOMBIA

Chapter
Junta National Liga Colombiana conta
la Epilepsia
Cap de Bolivar
Barrio Ternera
Calle 1a, El Eden, Y 5007 Cartagena

CROATIA

Chapter
University Hospital Center Rebro
Department of Paediatrics
Division of Nueropaediatrics
Kispaticeva 12Kispaticeva 12
1000 Zagreb

CUBA

Chapter
Sociedad de Neurosciencias de Cuba,
Seccion de Epilepsia
Hospital Psiquitrico de la Habana
Rpio Mazorra Ap9, Boyoros
Ciudad de las Habana, CP 19220

CZECH REPUBLIC

Chapter
Spolecnost "E"
Novodvorska 994
142 21 Prague 4

DENMARK

Chapter
Dansk Epilepsiforening
Kongensgade 68, 2. Tv.
DK-5000 Odense C

ECUADOR

Centro Nacional de Epilepsia APNE
Isla Marchena 300 y Los Granados
Casilla 17-15-221 C
Quito

ETHIOPIA

Epilepsy Support Association of
Ethiopia (ESAE)
CEO
P.O. Box 25516
Code 1000.Addis Ababa

FINLAND

Chapter
Epilepsialiitto
Malmin Kauppatie 26
FIN-00700
Helsinki

FRANCE

Chapter
A.I.S.P.A.C.E.
11 Avenue Kennedy
F-59800 Lille

GEORGIA

Chapter
Epilepsy and Environment Association
of Georgia
Department of Neurology
Tbilisi State Medical University
Jacob Nicoladze str. 6
app 22,380079 Tbilisi

GERMANY

Chapter
Deutsche Epilepsie Vereinigung
Zillestrasse 102
10585 Berlin

GHANA

Chapter
Ghana Epilepsy Association
c/o P.O. Box M230
Accra

GREECE

Chapter
Greek National Association Against
Epilepsy
Aghia Sophia Children's Hospital
Department of Neurology/
Neurophysiology
Athens 11527

GUATEMALA

Chapter
IBE Guatemalan *Chapter*
6a. Calle 2–48, Zona 1
Guatemala City

HUNGARY

Chapter
Hungarian Association of People Living
with Epilepsy
H-1028 Budapest
Hidegkuti ut 353

ICELAND

Chapter
LAUF, The Icelandic Epilepsy
Association
Postbox 5182
126 Reykjavik

INDIA

Chapter
Indian Epilepsy Association
Sannidhi
K-10/10, DLF Qutab Enclave II
Gurgaon – 122 022, via Delhi

INDONESIA

Chapter
PERPEI
Bagian Neurologi FKUI
Jl. Salemba 6
Jakarta Pusat

IRAN

Chapter
Iranian Epilepsy Association
P.O. Box 15655/199
Tehran

IRELAND

Chapter
Brainwave
Irish Epilepsy Association
249 Crumlin Road
Dublin 12

ISRAEL

Chapter
Israel Epilepsy Association
4 Avodat Yisrael St.
P.O. Box 91014
Jerusalem 91014

ITALY

Associazone Italiano contro l'Epilessia
(AICE)
via T Marino 7
20121 Milan

JAPAN

Japan Epilepsy Association
5F Zenkokuzaidan Building 2-2-8
Nishiwaseda Shinjuku-ku
Tokyo 162

KENYA

Chapter
Kenya Association for the Welfare of
Epileptics
P.O. Box 60790
Nairobi

KOREA

Chapter
Korean Epilepsy Association/Rose Club
110–021, Room No 301
Buwon Building
175–1 Buam-dong, Chongno-ku
Seoul

LITHUANIA

Chapter
Lithuanian Society of Epileptic Patients
and Their Sponsors
Kaunas Medical Univerity Hospital
Department of Neurosurgery
Eiveniu 2, LT-3007 Kaunas

MALAYSIA

Chapter
Persatuan Epilepsi Malaysia
Department of Neurology
Kuala Lumpur Hospital
Jalan Pahang 50586
Kuala Lumpur

MALTA

Chapter
Caritas Malta Epilepsy Association
5, Lion Street
Floriana

MEXICO

Chapter
Group "Acceptation" of Epileptics
Amsterdam 1928 No 19
Colonia Olimpica-Pedregal
Mexico 04710 DF

NEW ZEALAND

Chapter
Epilepsy New Zealand (ENZ)
National Office
P.O. Box 1074
Hamilton

NORWAY

Chapter
Norsk Epilepsiforbund
Storgt. 39
0182 Oslo

PERU

Chapter
Peruvian Association of Epilepsy
Jr. Castilla 678 E-101
Lima 32

POLAND

Chapter
Polish Epilepsy Association
ul. Fabryczna 57
15-482 Bialystok

PORTUGAL

Chapter
Portuguese League against Epilepsy
Servico de Neurologia
Hospital Santa Maria
Avenida Prof Egas Moniz
1649–035 Lisboa

SAUDI ARABIA

Chapter
Epilepsy Support and Information
Centre
P.O. Box 3354
MBC 76
Riyadh, 11211

SCOTLAND

Chapter
Epilepsy Action Scotland
48 Govan Road
Glasgow G51 1JL

SENEGAL

Chapter
Ligue Senegalaise contre l'Epilepsie
Clinique Neurologique
Centre Hospitalo–Universitaire de Fann
BP 5035, Dakar-Fann

SINGAPORE

Chapter
Singapore Epilepsy Foundation
2 Finlayson Green No 16/05
Asian Insurance Building
Singapore 049247

SLOVENIA

Chapter
Slovenian League Against Epilepsy
Institute of Clinical Neurophysiology
Hospital of Neurology, Medical Centre
SI-1525 Ljubljana

SOUTH AFRICA

Chapter
South African National Epilepsy
League
S.A.N.E.L.
P.O. Box 73
Observatory 7935
Capetown

SPAIN

Chapter
Asociacion Espnala de Ayda al
Epileptico
c/Berlin, 5, 40 Piso
28028 Madrid

SRI LANKA

Chapter
Epilepsy Association of Sri Lanka
10 Austin Place
Colombo 8

SWEDEN

Chapter
Swedish Epilepsy Association
P.O. Box 9514
102 74 Stockholm

SWITZERLAND

Chapter
Schweizerische Liga gegen Epilepsie
Dorfstrasse 2
Postfach 233
8712 Stafa/ZH, Zurich

TAIWAN

Chapter
Taiwan Epilepsy Association
P.O. Box 118-205
Taipei

TUNISIA

Chapter
Tunisian Epilepsy Association
Neurological Department
EPS Charles Nicolle
Tunis 1006

UNITED KINGDOM

Chapter
British Epilepsy Association
New Anstey House
Gate Way Drive
Yeadon, Leeds LS19 7XY

UNITED STATES

Chapter
Epilepsy Foundation
4351 Garden City Drive, 5th Floor
Landover, Maryland 20785

YUGOSLAVIA

Chapter
Jugoslovensko Drustvo za Epilepsiju
Slobadana Penezica-Krcuna 23
Beograd

ZIMBABWE

Epilepsy Support Foundation
P.O. Box 104, Avondale
Old General Hospital
Mazoe Street, Harare

Other International Epilepsy Resources

AUSTRIA

JOHANNA SCHALLMEINER
4674 Altenhof/Hausruck
Hueb 18
07735/73-13

INGE WEIDRINGER
4674 Altenhof
Hueb 14
07735/66-31-434

GERLINDE PRANDSTATTER
4020 Linz
Europastrabe 38
0732/38-75-74

PETER KOLLER
4100 Ottensheim
Stifterstrabe 34
07234/41-69

ALOIS U. UTA PUCHER
4774 St. Marienkirchen 143
07711/23-26

AUSTRALIA

MELBOURNE OFFICES
818 Burke Road
Camberwell 3124
(03) 9813-2866

WESTERN REGION OFFICE
41 Somerville Road
Yarraville 3013
(03) 9813-2866

WENDOUREE COMMUNITY CENTRE
1097 Howitt Street
Wendouree 3355
(053) 381-277

EAGLEHAWK AND LONG GULLY COMMUNITY HEALTH CENTRE
Seymoure Street
Eaglehawk 3556
(054) 468-800

ILLAWARRA COMMUNITY CENTRE
265 Pakington Street
Newtown 3220
(052) 231-645

MORWELL SCHOOL SUPPORT CENTRE
Harold Street
Morwell 3840
(051) 369-900

GOULBURN VALLEY COMMUNITY CARE CENTRE
162 Maude Street
Shepparton 3630
(058) 222-415

CANADA

EPILEPSY ASSOCIATION, METRO TORONTO
One St. Clair Avenue, East, Suite 500
Toronto ON M4T 2V7
(416) 964-9095

EPILEPSY ONTARIO
P.O. Box 58515
197 Sheppard Avenue East
North York, Ontario
M2N 6R7
(905) 764-5099

HAMILTON AND DISTRICT CHAPTER
92 King Street East, Suite 855
Hamilton, Ontario L8N 1A8
(905) 522-8487

OTTAWA-CARLETON CHAPTER
509-180 Metcalfe Street
Ottawa, Ontario
K2P 1P5
(613) 594-9255

ENGLAND

MERSEY REGION EPILEPSY ASSOCIATION
Glaxo Neurological Centre
Norton Street
Liverpool L3 8LR
0151 298 2666
0151 298 2333 Fax

GERMANY

GESCHAFTSSTELLE DER DEUTSCHEN SEKTION
der Internationalen Liga gegen Epilepsie
Frau Ingrid Kersten Havekost
Herforder Str. 5-7
D-33602 Bielefeld
49 521 12 41 92

HUNGARY

P. RAJNA
Hungarian Chapter of the
International League Against Epilepsy
P.O. Box 1
H-1261 Budapest 27

ICELAND

ICELANDIC EPILEPSY FOUNDATION (L.A.U.F.)
Laugarvegur 26
101 Reykjavik
P.O. Box 5182
125 Reykjavik
354-551-4570
354-551-4580 Fax

MALAYSIA

MALAYSIAN EPILEPSY SOCIETY
Neurology Department
Kuala Lumpur Hospital
50586 Kuala Lumpur
Malaysia
(603) 298-9845 Fax

SINGAPORE

THE EPILEPSY CARE GROUP
c/o Medical Alumni Association
2 College Road
Singapore 0316
Republic of Singapore
(epilepsy support group)

TAIWAN

DR. JING-JANE TSAI
President, Chinese Epilepsy Society
c/o Department of Neurology
National Cheng Kung University
Medical Center
138-Sheng-Li Road
Tainan 704
886 62 35 36 60

TURKEY

EPILEPSY SOCIETY OF TURKEY
Cigdem Ozkara, M.D.
I-7-C-27 7-8 Kisim Atakoy
34750 Istanbul
90212 55 90 815

UNITED KINGDOM

**BRITISH BRANCH OF THE
INTERNATIONAL LEAGUE
AGAINST EPILEPSY**
Dr. S. D. Shorvon
National Hospital for Nervous Diseases
Queen Square
London WC1N 3 BG
44 494 873 991

URUGUAY

DR. ALEJANDRO SCARAMELLI
Liga Uruguaya contra la Epilepsia
Hospital de Clinicas, Piso 2
Av. Italia s/n
11600 Montevideo
5982 471 221

Internet Resources

1. Epilepsy Foundation
   http://www.efa.org

2. National Institutes of Health, Women's Health Initiative
   http://www.healthtouch.com

3. Massachusetts General Hospital
   http://www.neuro-oas.mgh.harvard.edu/epilepsy

4. The Whole Brain Atlas
   http://www.med.harvard.edu/AANLIB/home.html

5. Epilepsy and Brain Mapping Program
   http://www.epipro.com/index.html

6. Mike Chee's Epilepsy Home Page
   http://www.home.earthlink.net/~mchee1/gnrchm2.htm

7. Washington University Comprehensive Epilepsy Program
   http://www.neuro.wustl.edu/epilepsy

8. Seizure-Alert Dogs
   http://www.vetmed.ufl.edu/ufmrg/dog/

9. KetoCal
   http://www.shsna.com

10. Cyberonics (vagal nerve stimulator)
    http://www.cyberonics.com

11. Andrew Wilner's Epilepsy Resources
    http://www.awilner.neurohub.net

12. Patient Assistance Programs
    http://www.needymeds.com

Glossary of Acronyms

ACTH:	adrenocorticotropic hormone
ADD:	attention deficit disorder
AED:	antiepileptic drug
AES:	American Epilepsy Society
AVM:	arteriovenous malformation
BECRS:	benign epilepsy of childhood with Rolandic spikes
CAT:	computerized axial tomography
CBC:	complete blood count
CBTL:	carbamazepine extended release (Carbatrol®)
CBZ:	carbamazepine (Tegretol®)
CCTV/EEG:	closed circuit television/electroencephalography
CNS:	central nervous system
CT:	computerized axial tomography (same as CAT)
EEG:	electroencephalograph
EF:	Epilepsy Foundation
EMU:	epilepsy monitoring unit
EPC:	epilepsia partialis continua
FBM:	felbamate
FDA:	Food and Drug Administration
GBP:	gabapentin (Neurontin®)
GTC:	generalized tonic clonic seizure (convulsion)
IRB:	institutional review board
IV:	intravenous
JME:	juvenile myoclonic epilepsy
LEV:	levetiracetam (Keppra®)
LFTS:	liver function tests
LTG:	lamotrigine (Lamictal®)
MEG:	magnetoencephalography
MRA:	magnetic resonance angiography
MRI:	magnetic resonance imaging
MRS:	magnetic resonance spectroscopy imaging

MTS:	mesial temporal sclerosis
OCBZ:	oxcarbazepine (Trileptal®)
PB:	phenobarbital
PDR:	*Physicians' Desk Reference*
PET:	positron emission tomography
PHT:	phenytoin (Dilantin®)
PI:	principal investigator
PRM:	primidone (Mysoline®)
SPECT:	single photon emission computed tomography
TGB:	tiagabine (Gabitril®)
TLE:	temporal lobe epilepsy
TPM:	topiramate (Topamax®)
VNS:	vagal nerve stimulator
VPA:	valproic acid (Depakene®)
VR:	vocational rehabilitation
ZNS:	zonisamide (Zonegran®)

MANAGED CARE

DM:	disease management
HMO:	health maintenance organization
IPA:	independent practice association
MCO:	managed care organization
PHO:	physician-hospital organization
PPO:	preferred provider organization

Glossary of Terms

Absence Seizure: A type of generalized seizure usually seen in children, characterized by staring, accompanied by a 3 per second spike and wave pattern on the electroencephalograph. These seizures respond well to medication and most children outgrow them.

Arteriovenous Malformation: A tangle of arteries and veins which can cause headaches, seizures, or bleeding in the brain. Often requires surgery.

Automatisms: Involuntary movements which accompany seizures, such as chewing, fumbling at a button, or pulling on clothes. Can occur in generalized or partial seizures.

Ataxia: A type of clumsiness, often the result of too much medication.

Aura: A warning that a seizure may begin, often described as a "funny feeling." An aura is actually a small seizure that may develop into a larger seizure, or disappear.

Benign Rolandic Epilepsy: Accounts for almost 25 percent of seizures appearing in children from age 5 to 14. Not always treated with medication, because seizures are typically outgrown by adolescence.

Catamenial: Related to a woman's monthly period.

Clonic Seizure: An epileptic seizure characterized by jerking.

Corpus Callosum: The white matter that connects the two hemispheres of the brain. A corpus callosotomy is an operation in which a part or all of this structure is cut, disconnecting the two hemispheres. This surgery is typically reserved for patients with intractable generalized epilepsy, such as the Lennox-Gastaut syndrome.

Computerized Axial Tomography: A CAT or CT scan. This type of x-ray uses a computer to assemble multiple images, producing a detailed picture of the skull and brain.

Comprehensive Epilepsy Center: A medical facility consisting of an epilepsy clinic and epilepsy monitoring unit staffed by neurologists, neurosurgeons, neuroradiologists, neuropsychologists, technologists, a clinical coordinator, and a social worker specially trained to help people with epilepsy. An epilepsy center also employs sophisticated technology such as magnetic resonance imaging, single photon emission computerized tomography, and positron emission tomography scans. (See Appendix D for a list of comprehensive epilepsy centers.)

Convulsion: A seizure characterized by stiffening of the body and jerking, excess salivation (foaming at the mouth), and loss of control of urine, followed by a period of confusion.

Déjà Vu: A psychic seizure that produces a false sense of familiarity, as if life is repeating itself.

Depth Electrode: A special electrode placed inside the brain through a small hole in the skull to locate a seizure focus.

Double Blind: A clinical trial in which medication is coded so that neither the doctor nor the patient knows whether placebo or active medication is being used.

Drop Attack: Often seen in Lennox-Gastaut syndrome, a type of seizure that causes the child to suddenly fall. May cause injuries of the face and head.

Electrode: A small metal contact attached to a wire designed to record brain waves from the scalp or inside the brain.

Electroencephalogram: A tracing of brain waves, used to search for epileptic spikes and abnormal slowing.

Encephalitis: An inflammation in the brain caused by infection. May be accompanied by seizures and result in epilepsy later in life.

Epilepsia Partialis Continua: A rare seizure type that consists of repeated jerking lasting long periods of time. Often seen in Rasmussen's encephalitis.

Epileptic Focus: The site in the brain where a seizure begins.

Epileptologist: A neurologist with special training who treats patients with epilepsy.

Febrile Seizure: A seizure caused by a high fever in children under the age of five. Most of these children do not develop epilepsy.

Fit: A seizure.

Generalized Seizure: A seizure that affects both hemispheres of the brain.

Grand Mal Seizure: A convulsion.

Grid: An array of electrodes placed on the brain to locate a seizure focus or map speech.

Half-Life: The time required for half the amount of drug to disappear from the body.

Health Management Organization: Members of this type of health plan pay a fixed monthly fee, regardless of their health care needs. They must use certain doctors and hospitals. Expensive tests and services can be more difficult to obtain.

Hemispherectomy: A type of epilepsy surgery in which one of the hemispheres of the brain is removed or disconnected. Can be extremely helpful in controlling seizures in appropriate patients.

Hypsarrhythmia: A specific pattern of irregular high amplitude slow waves and spikes on the electroencephalogram seen in West's syndrome.

Indemnity Insurance: Allows purchasers to choose their own doctor. Pays a percentage of the total bill after a deductible.

Infantile Spasms: A type of seizure that occurs in infants, characterized by frequent jerks of the body. Part of West's syndrome.

Intractable: Refers to seizures that cannot be stopped by medication.

Intravenous: Medications or fluids administered through a needle inside a vein.

Lennox-Gastaut Syndrome: A type of epilepsy occurring in infancy and early childhood characterized by frequent seizures and multiple seizure types. These children have mental retardation and slow spike and wave complexes on their electroencephalograms. This type of epilepsy is extremely difficult to control.

Liver Function Test Abnormality: An elevation of liver enzymes, which can be caused by antiepileptic medications. This is a common finding on blood tests and not a cause for concern unless the level is very high.

Low White Count: An abnormality detected on a complete blood count (CBC), often a side effect of antiepileptic medications. Rarely of clinical significance.

Magnetic Resonance Imaging: A scan that uses an enormous magnet instead of x-rays to form an extremely detailed image of the brain.

Magnetic Resonance Angiography: A magnetic scan of the blood vessels of the brain. Does not require any contrast material (dye).

Magnetic Resonance Spectroscopy: A new method of measuring brain metabolism using a magnetic scanner to identify a seizure focus.

Magnetoencephalography: An experimental device that measures minute magnetic fields produced by ionic currents in the brain; may help localize an epileptic focus.

Medicaid: A state-administered program of federal financial assistance primarily for families with children, the aged, blind, and disabled.

Medicare: A federally funded health insurance program primarily for people age 65 and older and the disabled.

Meningitis: An inflammation of the coverings of the brain.

Monotherapy: Single drug treatment for epilepsy.

Myoclonus: A sudden muscle jerk of the body. Can be seen in a number of different epilepsy syndromes.

Neuron: A nerve cell. Billions of neurons interact to make up a working brain. Epileptic discharges are produced when groups of neurons misfire.

Nystagmus: Bouncing eye movements, often the result of medication toxicity.

Open Label: A clinical trial in which the name and dosage of the investigational drug are known to the investigator and patient.

Partial Seizure: A seizure that begins in a specific location in the brain, such as the temporal lobe.

Partial Complex Seizure: A seizure that begins in a specific location in the brain and alters consciousness, causing confusion.

Partial Simple Seizure: A seizure that begins in a specific location in the brain but does not alter consciousness. It may produce an abnormal sensation, such as an unpleasant smell, or a motor movement, such as jerking of an arm.

Petit Mal Seizure: Same as absence seizure.

Placebo: An inactive substance sometimes used as a basis for comparison when new drugs are tested.

Polytherapy: Treatment with multiple drugs.

Positron Emission Tomography: A scan that uses an injection of radioactive tracer to measure brain metabolism in an effort to locate the seizure focus. Often part of the evaluation before seizure surgery.

Postictal: The period immediately after a seizure.

Preferred Provider Organization: An insurance plan that allows members to use specified doctors in a discounted fee for service arrangement.

Protocol: The specific manner in which a clinical trial is conducted.

Pseudoseizures: Clinically resemble epileptic seizures but without epileptic discharges from the brain. Also called psychogenic or nonepileptic seizures, most often caused by severe psychosocial stress.

Rasmussen's Encephalitis: A type of chronic, progressive brain inflammation that produces uncontrolled seizures. May be successfully treated by hemispherectomy.

Single Photon Emission Computerized Tomography: A scan that uses an injection of a radioactive tracer to measure blood flow in the brain. Typically two SPECT scans are done, one during a seizure and one in between seizures. SPECT scans can help identify a seizure focus in preparation for seizure surgery.

Spike: A characteristic finding on the electroencephalograph in patients with epilepsy. A spike is the result of an abnormal synchronized electrical discharge in a population of neurons.

Status Epilepticus: A condition of recurrent seizures on the same day or prolonged seizures requiring immediate medical attention.

Telemetry: Continuous monitoring of the electroencephalogram, often with video.

Temporal Lobe: A part of the brain important in memory and controlling speech. Often the site of the epileptic focus.

Therapeutic Range: A guide, and only a guide, for antiepileptic drug levels. Patients often require more or less medication to control their seizures than suggested by the therapeutic range listed on the laboratory report.

Todd's Paralysis: A temporary weakness of an arm, leg, or other body part after a seizure.

Tonic seizure: An epileptic seizure characterized by stiffening.

Toxicity: An undesirable effect of medication such as drowsiness, dizziness, trouble walking, or difficulty concentrating.

Tuberous Sclerosis: An inherited disorder, typically with mental retardation, abnormalities of the brain, skin, and other organs, and seizures. Half of these patients will have infantile spasms.

Vagal Stimulator: A device designed to control seizures, similar to a cardiac pacemaker, but with the electrode attached to the vagus nerve in the neck.

Wada Test: Not an abbreviation, but named after its developer, Dr. Jun Wada. This is an injection into the carotid artery of amobarbital (Amytal®), used to determine the location of the brain's speech center and test memory prior to epilepsy surgery.

West Syndrome: A type of epilepsy in infants characterized by abrupt spasms of the body that usually occur in clusters, mental retardation, and a recognizable pattern on the electroencephalograph called hypsarrhythmia.

Bibliography

Additional Information

1. *Managing Your Epilepsy.* Ilo E. Leppik, Handbooks in HealthCare Co, Newtown, Pennsylvania, 2000.

2. *The Epilepsy Diet Treatment: An Introduction to the Ketogenic Diet,* 3rd edition, J. Freeman, M. Kelly, and J. Freeman, Demos Vermande, New York, 1999.

3. *Health Insurance: How to Get It, Keep It, or Improve What You've Got,* 2nd edition, Robert Enteen, Demos Vermande, New York, 1996.

4. *Clinical Trials: What You Should Know Before Volunteering to Be a Research Subject,* J. Joseph Giffels, Demos Vermande, New York, 1996.

5. *Living Well with Epilepsy,* Robert J. Gumnit, 2nd edition. Demos Vermande, New York, 1996.

6. *Your Child and Epilepsy,* Robert J. Gumnit, Demos Vermande, New York, 1995.

7. *Epilepsy A to Z: A Glossary of Epilepsy Terminology,* P. Kaplan, P. Loiseau, R. Fisher, P. Jallon, Demos Vermande, New York, 1995.

8. *A Guide to Understanding and Living with Epilepsy,* Orrin Devinsky, F.A. Davis Co., Philadelphia, 1994.

9. *Seizures and Epilepsy in Childhood: A Guide for Parents,* J. Freeman, E. Vining, D. Pillas, The Johns Hopkins University Press, Baltimore, 1991.

10. *Children with Epilepsy, A Parents' Guide,* edited by Helen Reisner, Woodbine House, Rockville, 1988.

Other Books of Interest

1. *The Brainstorms Healer,* Steven C. Schachter, A. James Rowan (eds.), Lippincott-Raven, Philadelphia, 1998.

2. *The Brainstorms Family,* Steven C. Schachter, Georgia D. Montouris, John M. Pellock (eds.), Lippincott-Raven, Philadelphia, 1996.

3. *Miles to Go Before I Sleep, My Grateful Journey Back from the Hijacking of Egypt Air Flight* 648, Jackie Nink Pflug, Hazelden Foundation, Center City, Minnesota, 1996.

4. *Equal Partners, A Physician's Call for a New Spirit of Medicine,* Jody Heymann, Little, Brown and Company, Boston, 1995.

5. *Epilepsy, I Can Live With That! Writings by People with Epilepsy*, Sue Goss (ed.), Epilepsy Foundation of Victoria, Inc., Victoria, Australia, 1995.

6. *The Brainstorms Companion, Epilepsy in Our View*, Steven C. Schachter (ed.), Lippincott-Raven, Philadelphia, 1995.

7. *Epilepsy: A New Approach*, Adrienne Richard and Joel Reiter, Walker and Company, New York, 1995.

8. *The Falling Sickness: A History of Epilepsy from the Greeks to the Beginnings of Modern Neurology*, Oswei Temkin, The Johns Hopkins University Press, Baltimore, 1994.

9. *Brainstorms: Epilepsy in Our Words, Personal Accounts of Living with Seizures*, Steven C. Schachter (ed.), Lippincott-Raven, Philadelphia, 1993.

10. *Mom, I Have a Staring Problem*, Marian and Tiffany Buckel, Marian Buckel, Bradenton, 1992.

11. *Embrace the Dawn: One Woman's Story of Triumph Over Epilepsy*, Andrea Davidson, Sylvan Creek Press, McCall, 1989.

12. *A Bomb in the Brain: A Heroic Tale of Science, Surgery, and Survival*, Steve Fishman, Avon Books, New York, 1988.

Afterword

I hope you enjoyed reading this book. Now that you know the answers to these 199 questions, you can manage your epilepsy with greater understanding and success.

Advances in epilepsy treatment continue at a rapid pace.

Because of continued progress in the treatment of epilepsy, another updated edition of *Epilepsy: 199 Answers* is inevitable if the information is to stay current. If you have questions that you think should be included in future editions, please send them to my attention at:

Demos
386 Park Avenue South
Suite 201
New York, NY 10016

In the meantime, work closely with your doctor, take advantage of the many helpful resources listed in this book, and good luck in controlling your seizures!

Index

Related Titles

Growing Up with Epilepsy: A Practical Guide for Parents
by Lynn Bennett Blackburn, Ph.D.

This book was developed to provide you with an "owner's manual" that will help you negotiate the unique challenges of childhood epilepsy. It provides the basic tools for understanding epilepsy, behavior management, and school programs for children with epilepsy. • 2003; ISBN: 1-888799-74-9; Price $19.95; Length est. 156 pages

The Ketogenic Diet: A Treatment for Epilepsy, Third Edition
by John M. Freeman, M.D., Jennifer B. Freeman and Millicent T. Kelly, R.D., L.D.

The Ketogenic Diet is the only book devoted exclusively to the Ketogenic diet. It has all the facts about the Ketogenic diet, numerous quotes from parents showing what the experience is really like, and thirty-five clear tested sample recipes. Every doctor and dietitian, who treats children with epilepsy, and every parent of a child with epilepsy, should read this book. • 1999; ISBN: 1-888799-39-0; Price: $24.95; 1-888799-39-0

Your Child and Epilepsy by Robert J. Gumnit, M.D.

Here is a wealth of practical information to help parents understand their childrens' epilepsy, suggestions on how to evaluate health care, to find better care if necessary, and advice on how to help children with epilepsy to develop self-confidence, and self-motivation. • 1995; ISBN: 0-939957-76-0; Price: $24.95; 256 pages

**Insurance Solutions–Plan Well, Live Better: A Workbook for People
with Chronic Illnesses or Disabilities** by Laura D. Cooper Esq.

Packed with ideas and strategies, this handy guide will help you find and purchase insurance that a typical insurance company might not make available to a disabled person. You will also find suggestions for obtaining insurance when traditional sources appear to be closed. • 2002; ISBN: 1-888799-55-2; Price: $24.95; 192 pages

**Health Insurance Resource Manual: Options for People with a Chronic
Disease or Disability** by Dorothy E. Northrop, MSW, ACSW and Stephen Cooper

This book was developed to assist people with disabilities and chronic health conditions to understand the health care system and maximize their rights and entitlements within that system. • 2003; ISBN: 1-888799-69-2; Price: $24.95; 186 Pages

To order call Demos Medical Publishing, Inc. at 1-800-532-8663
or visit our website at http://www.demosmedpub.com

Notes